WHY MY HEART IS PURPLE

250TH U.S. ARMY BIRTHDAY EDITION

MATTHEW SIMS

WHY MY HEART IS PURPLE

by Matthew Sims
Copyright © 2024
All rights reserved.

Library of Congress Number: 2024946580
International Standard Book Number: 978-1-60126-953-9

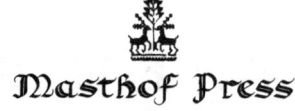

219 Mill Road | Morgantown, PA 19543-9516
www.Masthof.com

TABLE OF CONTENTS

The Combat Medic Prayer iv
Endorsements v
Introduction ix
Dedication x
Bio xi

SECTION 1

Chapter 1: Wounded But Willing 1
Chapter 2: Fast Forward 11 Years 6
Chapter 3: The Day I Earned the Title "DOC" 7
Chapter 4: To Hurt or To Heal 15
Chapter 5: Our Iraqi Brothers 18
Chapter 6: Baby Boom! 21
Chapter 7: Dove for Dinner 26
Chapter 8: Right Place Right Time to Save a Life 29
Chapter 9: Soldier's Medal 31
Chapter 10: Making an Impact 34
My Favorite Patriotic Speech 38

SECTION 2

Those Who Gave It All 44

Epilogue 160
Editor's Note 161

THE COMBAT MEDIC PRAYER

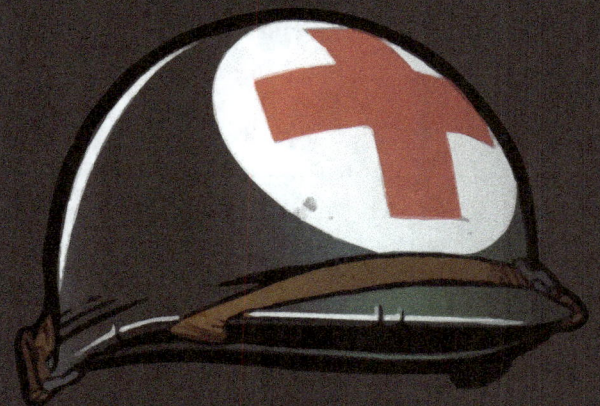

Oh, Lord, I ask for your divine strength to meet the demands of my profession. Help me to be the finest medic, both technically and tactically. If I am called to the battlefield, give me the courage to conserve our fighting forces by providing medical care to all who are in need.

If I am called to a mission of peace, give me the strength to lead by caring for those who need my assistance.

Finally, Lord, help me to take care of my own spiritual, physical, and emotional needs. Teach me to trust in your presence and never-failing love.

AMEN

ENDORSEMENTS

Operation Second Chance, Inc.

As the Founder and CEO of Operation Second Chance, Inc., I am delighted to write this letter in support of Matthew Sims, a three-time Purple Heart recipient whose bravery and resilience shine through in his profoundly moving book, *Why My Heart Is Purple*.

Matthew's narrative is not just a memoir; it is a captivating page-turner that skillfully combines raw courage with heartfelt emotion. Through *Why My Heart Is Purple*, Matthew Sims offers readers a deeply personal journey that resonates on multiple levels. His ability to convey the realities of his experiences as a combat medic, is both poignant and enlightening.

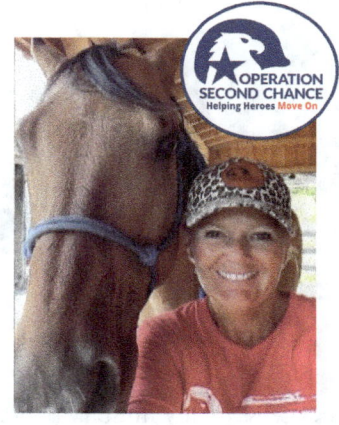

Cindy McGrew with Cactus, one of the beloved horses at Heroes Ridge Veterans' Retreat, Raven Rock, MD.

What sets Matthew's book apart is its ability to engage readers on a visceral level. Each page is infused with the reality of war zones as a combat medic tends to his brothers in arms. His passion as a medic and authenticity is what keeps the reader invested from start to finish. It is rare to encounter a work that educates the reader on the reality of war. It accomplishes all of this effortlessly.

I have no doubt that Matthew Sims' powerful storytelling and profound insights will leave a lasting impact on its readers. His perspective as a decorated veteran adds a unique dimension to the narrative, making *Why My Heart Is Purple* a must-read for anyone seeking to understand what happens in a combat zone. I wholeheartedly recommend Matthew Sims and his exceptional book, as a testament to bravery, resilience, and the power of storytelling. I am confident that Matthew's work will resonate deeply with a wide audience.

Thank you for considering my recommendation.

With a grateful heart,
Cindy McGrew

General Tommy Franks Leadership Institute and Museum

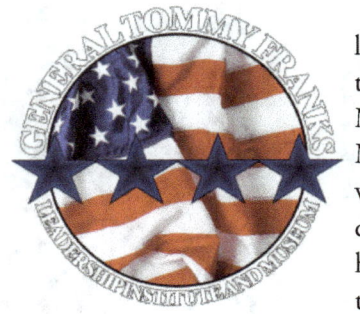

I am honored to endorse Matt Sims' latest book, *Why My Heart is Purple*. During the partnership my Leadership Institute and Museum has had with him for many years, Matt represents the best example of an individual who is a true "American Patriot." He deeply cares for our country and everyone he comes into contact with—especially on the battlefield.

Combat medics are crucial to the success of any military operation, and Matt has proved that many times. His is a story that must be told—so glad it is being published. We all must not forget the sacrifices these American heroes made in supporting their fellow troopers.

Our museum has several incredibly unique exhibits that tell the story of many brave individuals. We are fortunate to have Matt's helmet he was wearing when shot in Iraq along with a piece of shrapnel that was pulled from his lung. This display exemplifies what our soldiers experience on the battlefield and is of great interest.

Matt has also been very involved in several of our programs: the grand marshal for our annual "Celebration of Freedom Parade;" spoke to our "4 Star Leadership Program" and volunteered with several of our functions. We are truly fortunate to have Matt involved. It really is having a lasting impact.

His new book will be a welcome addition to the many untold stories about true heroes who fought and died defending this great country.

Respectfully,

Tommy Franks
General, retired

Mid America Veterans Museum

It is an honor and privilege to endorse Matt Sims' latest book, *Why My Heart Is Purple*. During my tenure as president of the Mid America Veterans Museum, I've had the privilege to utilize Matt as a resource, representative, speaker, and share his story. His is a story of sacrifice and devotion—to duty and others. Combat medics and corpsmen are unsung heroes and represent a unique and special commitment to their brothers and sisters in arms. They touch countless lives and bravely serve in mostly adverse conditions.

Our museum's mission is unique in that we collect veterans' stories, assist in the writing of their story, preserve stories, and share them. Virtually all our visitors to our museum hear Matt's story and visit his display. Our display includes Matt's shrapnel shredded uniform, when his ambulance hit a roadside bomb, earning his first of three Purple Hearts. We also have a special collection of letters written to Matt from comrades, friends, and parents expressing their gratitude. When you read the letters, you learn, medics and corpsman needn't wonder if they made a difference in this world.

We must never forget the sacrifices of our veterans. While some gave all, all gave some. Matt's book contains stories about heroes, written by a true American hero and patriot. It is paramount we preserve and share the stories of our veterans for future generations. The cost of war is high, and it is important to help the public understand that our veterans bear visible and invisible scars. Stories like Matt's must be shared and told. We are grateful and proud to display his story.

To read Matt's story in the museum, visit www.mavm.org.

Sincerely,

Jim Higgins
Former President, Mid America Veterans Museum
Operations Manager, Historian

Matt's Commanding Officer

Matt's book *Why My Heart Is Purple* is just the tip of the iceberg. Matt somehow manages to consistently be where he needs to be—and then—has the courage to do what needs to be done. Always!

I once joked that I wasn't sure I wanted to hang out with him since people near him often seemed to get hurt and be in danger. Then I realized that those who got hurt near Matt were most likely to survive. I have known him for almost a decade now and had the privilege of working alongside him for two of those years. During our time together I had almost daily interaction with him as well as being privy to a slew of Matt Sims stories as recited by Matt himself, but more importantly and frequently by those he served and assisted in life.

While serving with him, a week rarely passed that I did not receive an email or phone call reciting what he had done for someone. He took an aging veteran he came across in a parking lot to buy a new battery for his vehicle; he changed a flat tire; he witnessed a catastrophic accident on the highway and saved a man's life; he saved a woman's life on a lake dinner cruise.

There is no place I would rather be than alongside Matthew Sims. Matthew Sims is a true servant....

- John A. Urciuoli
COL. (R) U.S. Army

INTRODUCTION

Why My Heart Is Purple *is my Special Edition book commemorating June 14, 2025—the United States Army's 250th Birthday.*

The U.S. Army traces its origins back to June 14, 1775, when the Continental Congress authorized the enlistment of expert riflemen to serve the United Colonies for one year. This action led to the creation of the Continental Army, which eventually evolved into today's U.S. Army.

George Washington was appointed as the first Commander in Chief of this newly established force, marking a pivotal moment in American history.

I am proud to have been part of this noble institution. Serving as a Soldier has been an honor, and I am grateful for the opportunities and experiences it has provided. The sense of purpose and commitment to something greater than oneself is a cornerstone of Army life.

For me, the Army's birthday is not just a celebration of its history, but also a reflection on the personal journeys of every Soldier who has served. It is a time to honor the friendships, the sacrifices, and the enduring spirit of service that defines the Army. Here's to the Army's legacy and to all those who have served and continue to serve with pride and dedication.

Why My Heart Is Purple brings you one Combat Medic's true historical account of a Soldier at war. As well it is a tribute to 219 military medical personnel who lost their lives trying to save others. All Soldiers in this book have earned the Purple Heart.

- Matthew Sims

DEDICATION

This book is dedicated to the men and women of the United States Army Medical Department. Without each Doctor, Nurse, Medic and Technician that helped me through my combat injuries I would not be here today to write this book. Every one of them touched my life in a positive way and helped me recover from my wounds of war.

I also dedicate this book to my parents, Bill and Shirley Sims, for raising me right and building me into the man I am today.

Finally, I dedicate this book to my wife Tina; without her and her love and support I could not have made it through the hard times.

Tina, "I love you more than anything in the world."

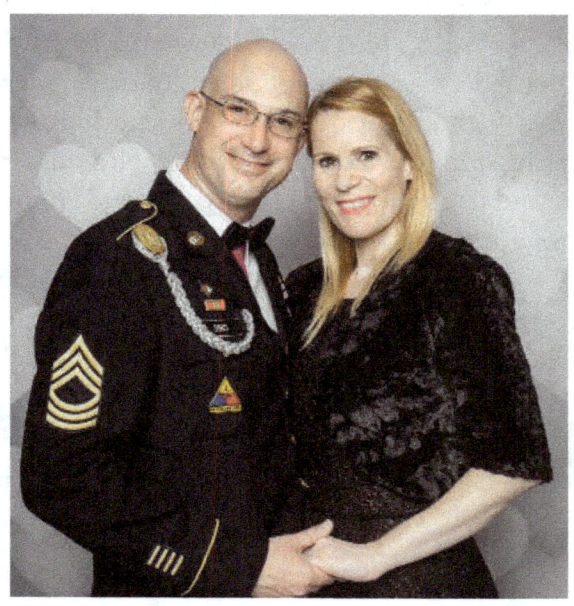

BIO

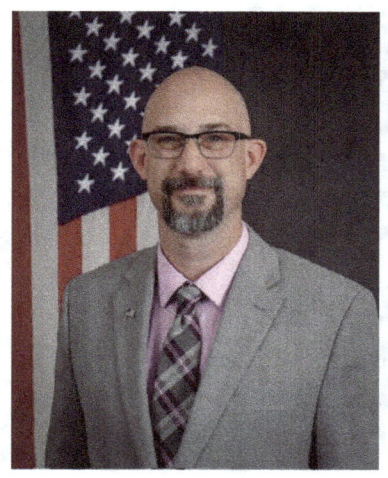

Master Sergeant (R) Matthew W. Sims was born in St. Charles, Missouri. He graduated from St. Charles High School in 1997. At the age of 17 he required parental permission to pursue his greatest desire to serve his country. June 14th, 1997, Matt enlisted in the Army and attended Basic Combat Training at Fort Leonard Wood, Missouri. Following basic training, he attended Advanced Individual Training at Fort Sam Houston, Texas to become a Combat Medic (68W). He holds degrees conferred in Health Science and Healthcare Administration from Purdue University and has been through the military professional training offered to enlisted service members such as Senior and Advanced Leader Courses.

Master Sergeant (R) Sims' assignments have varied throughout his military career: serving as a Combat Medic in Air Defense Artillery; Field Artillery; Engineer Units in Germany; and two Armor Cavalry Regiments and Armor Battalions in Colorado and Kansas.

He has held operational leadership roles in tactical organizations. As well, he has served in multiple roles at military health clinics and hospitals in Virginia and Oklahoma, taking care of both military Soldiers and their family members. Sims also held a special assignment in the 30th Medical Brigade as an Inspector General in Germany.

He deployed as a Combat Medic, supporting a multitude of military engagements such as **Operation Desert Tempest** (Saudi Arabia); **Operation Iraqi Freedom** (Iraq); **Operation Enduring Freedom** (Afghanistan), and **Operation New Dawn** (Iraq, Kuwait). While deployed in support of Operation Iraqi Freedom III, Master Sergeant Sims was wounded three separate times in one combat tour.

His wounds included a broken neck, fractured skull, fractured femur, collapsed lung, and shrapnel wounds to his left leg, where he would ultimately be awarded three Purple Hearts.

Upon retirement, Master Sergeant Sims' military decorations included: ***Legion of Merit; two Soldiers Medals; three Purple Hearts; two Meritorious Service Medals; four Army Commendation Medals; Army Good Conduct Medal with seven knots; Military Outstanding Volunteer Service Medal; Combat Medic Badge and Expert Field Medical Badge.***

He officially retired from active-duty service in March 2019 and currently resides in Elgin, Oklahoma, with his wife, Tina.

Matthew is currently employed by the Department of Defense as the Administrator of the Health Care Facility at Fort Sill, Oklahoma.

SECTION 1

FOREWORD

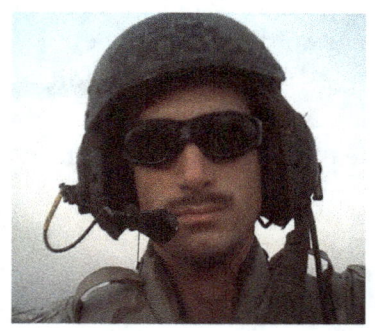

I want to thank Masthof Press for the opportunity to bring my story to the American public. When I wrote this book, I never thought it would actually be published one day. That day has come. Take and read!

I served 23 years as a Combat Medic in the U.S. Army and earned three Purple Hearts during my last tour in Iraq. The Purple Heart is given to service members who are wounded or killed in combat. The Purple Heart is the oldest military medal and was designed by General George Washington himself.

I often find myself reflecting on what it means to receive this venerable medal, a symbol that resonates deep within the hearts of Americans. The Purple Heart is not just an ornament or decoration, it is a tribute to sacrifice, to the valor of those who have given something of themselves for something greater than themselves.

It is a mark of courage, fortitude, and an unbreakable commitment to the principles that make our nation strong. When I think of the Purple Heart, I see faces of friends and comrades, some of whom are no longer with us. I feel the weight of their dedication and the warmth of their patriotism, a fire that burns eternally bright, fueled by love for our great country.

I remember the brave men and women who have spilled their blood on distant battlefields, those who returned home with wounds seen and unseen, and those who paid the ultimate price. Their sacrifices have shaped our history, strengthened our resolve, and defined our character as a nation.

But honoring them is not only about looking back, but it is also a reminder to look forward, to recognize the resilience and commitment that lives within us all. It is a call to nurture the values of compassion, integrity, and determination, which are the backbone of our community and our county.

Their sacrifice is not in vain. Their pain is our shared responsibility, and their triumph is our collective pride. They are an inspiration, a beacon of what it means to be American, and their legacy will live on through the ages.

May we never forget what the Purple Heart symbolizes and always strive to live up to the ideals it represents. Section 2 will help tell the story of 219 of these brave men & women.

Chapter 1

WOUNDED BUT WILLING

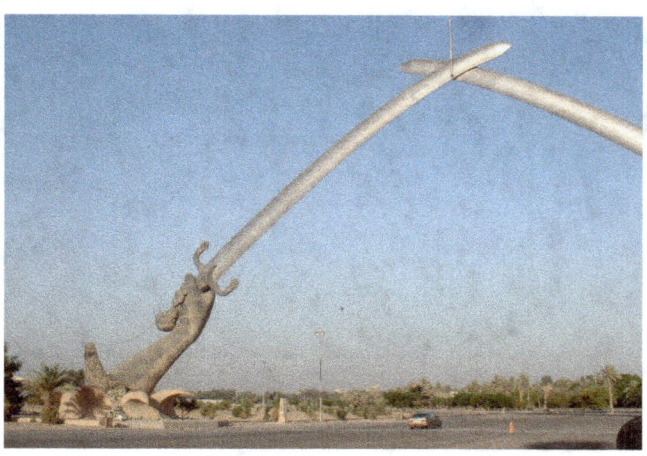

Entering Baghdad

I want to start by telling a story. This story is about a young Combat Medic. The story begins in Iraq in 2005. This young medic is deployed with an Armor Battalion, as the Senior Medic for Bravo Company. This is the medic's first deployment to Iraq, and he is so motivated to try out his new leadership skills and his medic talents—he is motivated to go out onto the battlefield to save lives!

The first few months of his tour go by without incident. He goes on numerous patrols, mounted and dismounted. And luckily, he has not had to crack open his freshly-stocked aid bag.

But that quickly changes on 2 February 2005, about 30 minutes into a convoy patrol with his unit. The convoy consists of two M1A1 Abrams Tanks and a Medical 113 Track Ambulance under his command. As if out of nowhere, the ear-piercing sound of an IED explosion is screaming through the air with hot shrapnel piercing like a tin can ripping through the armor of the ambulance. The hot smell burns his nostrils.

The hot shrapnel pierces the vehicle, striking the medic on his right side, ripping through his vest. After realizing what had happened, he sees the blood, he is bleeding with severe pain shooting through his right torso. He is HIT!

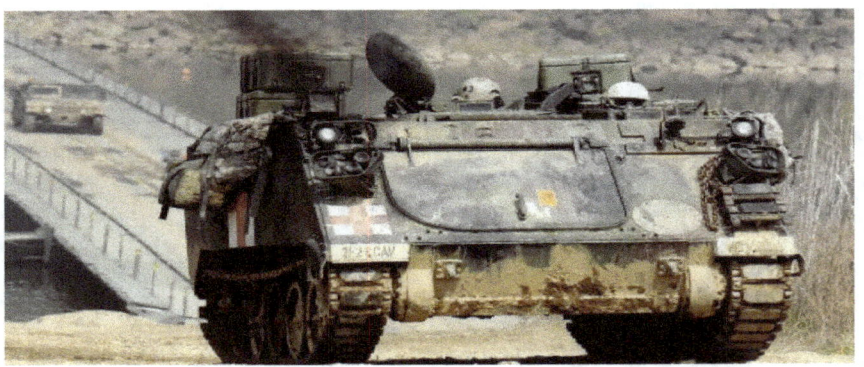

M113 Track Ambulance Sims was riding in when hit.

The driver of the vehicle was able to move out of the blast zone. That is when the medic realizes he has a collapsed lung. Being that he is the only medic on the patrol, he knows he alone must not panic and rely on his combat lifesaver's training to treat his own critical wounds. His mind rapidly searches for the procedures. Every second counts now! Then his training kicks into gear. The medic knows that if the pressure is not relieved from his lung, he will eventually lose his ability to breathe.

A young combat lifesaver comes up from the patrol, "*Doc what do I need to do?*"

"Do you remember the needle decompression technique you learned in the combat lifesaver course? You are going to have to do that to me," he instructs.

Without hesitation the Soldier prepares his 14-gauge needle and prepares to stick it between the medic's ribs. Steeling himself, the medic knows what is about to happen, and bares down for the pain. The needle hits its mark, and the medic instantly can breathe easy again.

Later, he hears the blades of a Blackhawk helicopter approaching. A welcome sound as he is loaded and evacuated to the Ballad hospital, where his treatment is continued. The next day the battalion commander and company commander came to visit him. After a long talk, the conversation turns to going home. The medic tells his command team that, if possible, he wants to stay and recover in Iraq. With the approval of his command and his doctors the medic is allowed to stay. After spending 37 days in the hospital the medic is released back to his unit.

After arriving back to his unit, he takes a few weeks to relax, but wants desperately to get back out on patrols. His unit is taking heavy casualties and he wants to get back to what he loves—being a combat medic—his passion is strong!

Two weeks later he finds himself on another patrol. This time he is pondering! The medic wants to provide medical coverage and decides maybe there would be a little place for him in the M1 tank. He finds himself that little place in the gunner's hatch of the lead tank and settles in. Driving down the main service route (MSR) Tamp, it's a cool uneventful evening, and the patrol is on its way back to Camp Taji, when the medic starts to see flashes in the distance.

Later he finds out that those flashes were from an enemy weapon, and that the bullet struck him directly in the front of his helmet. The force of the impact knocked him unconscious, and he fell into the turret of the tank. He wakes up 20 minutes later lying in the middle of the road with his entire team protecting him.

He hears the familiar sounds of helicopter rotor blades and thinks to himself, "I have bought myself another trip to the Ballad hospital."

But this time he has no pain; he just feels disoriented. After spending a few days at the hospital, it is determined that his neck is broken and he has a small skull fracture, and to add to that also a fracture in his left leg. Luckily, the neck fracture is minor. Well at least as minor as a broken neck can be.

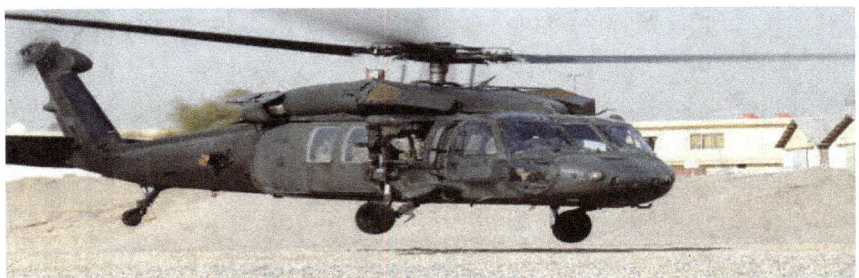

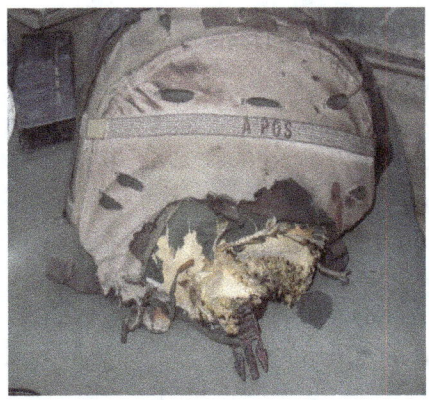

Sims' shattered helmet and the helicopter that carried him back to Ballad hospital.

Once again, his command team comes to visit, and once again the conversation turns to going home. The medic asks his commander again if he could stay and recover in Iraq. And once again with the approval from his doctor the medic is allowed to stay.

After eight weeks of recovery, he is released back to his unit. He immediately starts to go on patrols again. This time he is on a dismounted foot patrol with his platoon. About 30 minutes into the patrol the element starts to take mortar fire. And before anyone can take cover one of the platoon members is struck in the abdomen by mortar shrapnel. The medic instantly starts treating his fellow platoon member. But before he can finish treatment, another mortar round hits near them.

The medic is struck in the leg by mortar shrapnel. The shrapnel entered the front of his leg and exited the side. Although the medic is wounded, he continues to treat his casualty.

While he was treating the abdominal wound, two combat life-savers treat his leg wound by putting on a tourniquet. Because the platoon is still under enemy fire the evacuation helicopter will not enter the area. This is a high danger zone of combat. The decision is made to hoof it back to base.

The medic and the soldier with the abdominal wound are able to make the 25-minute walk back to the FOB, where they are both evacuated to the *familiar* Ballad hospital. Once again, the medic's command come to visit, and again he asks to stay and recover in Iraq, and once again permission is granted. Luckily, there are only a few more months left on the deployment and after being wounded three times the medic is restricted to the base and finishes his deployment working in the Aid Station.

Chapter 2

FAST FORWARD 11 YEARS

Now I will fast forward 11 years. The medic has now almost fully recovered from his injuries. Although there will always be lingering pain. In 2016 the same medic is diagnosed not once, but twice with cancer. He undergoes numerous rotations of radiation treatment and chemotherapy. For six months he fights cancer and is finally told the magic words every cancer patient wants to hear. *You are cancer free.*

The story you just read is about me. Although the story is about me, the legacy of it is not. The legacy is about my parents, who raised me to be a good person. It is about my wife who has supported me through all the long deployments, field training exercises and late nights that go along with being a Soldier. It is about my grandma who had hundreds of people praying for me. It is about my grandpa, Calvin, who died the day before I was shot in the head and was there protecting me. It is about Drill Sergeant Williams who taught me how to be a Soldier. It is about my first squad leader who took me under his wing and showed me what right looked like. It is about PFC Clark, the combat lifesaver who treated my collapsed lung. It is about SPC Johnson who put the tourniquet on my leg. It is about Dr. Timms who allowed me to stay in Iraq. It is about Army Medicine as a whole. Because without Army Medicine and each and every medic, nurse, and doctor that helped me along the way I would not be alive today to write this book. In the end it is about every service member who has come before me and every service member who has paid the ultimate sacrifice. Because without that sacrifice, America would not be the same. Freedom isn't free.

CHAPTER 3

THE DAY I EARNED THE TITLE "DOC"

I am trying to write something I have not been brave enough to put into words before. To feel something new. This is the first time I can verbalize and share with painful, haunting memory.

My mind is saying, "*Try to keep James alive by remembering him.*"

War is a place where boys become men. *The unfortunate truth is, not every man comes home.* This story is my point of view from the day one man took his last breath.

In response to frequent insurgent encounters, our task force was given a mission. We had been doing frequent patrols through the village of Lutafia, Iraq, and it is not uncommon to have a few shots taken at us each time. IEDs are being found more often in the area and reports of a local insurgent leader being in the area is confirmed. Over the period of a week, "Operation Smack Down" was supposed to weed out the local insurgents. The plan is not to go looking for a fight, but to bring the fight to us *on our terms*. Just two days prior, we had conducted a series of raids within the village and had acquired the high-level target we had been searching for. No casualties had been sustained from our side, and our team was on a kind of high, after a successful mission. We now had a day to rest, refit, and prepare for what was to come next.

That morning started just like every other day. We wake up early on the morning of the 13th. To be honest, I do not think I ever really slept; I am sure I am not the only one. The air is still warm as we gather for our pre-mission briefing and morning prayer. The moon is still hanging overhead as we receive the information about today's mission. We have no idea what this day will bring.

There is an intense sense of anxiety that we all seem to share. It seems to hang in the air almost palpable. Huddled there in the dark, we pray the Lord's Prayer as we have done so many times before. It has become so repetitive, yet we had not lost its meaning. Asking for protection in the face of adversity just became commonplace.

"*Amen,*" echoes out of the darkness.

As we utter the last words of the prayer, there are shouts of excitement. The sound of Soldiers getting themselves hyped for the mission that lies ahead, not unlike the locker room of a football team right before a big game. I take a moment and look at all the faces of these young men.

These men had become my family; they are my responsibility. I am their medic. We plan for the worst but hope for the best, I reflect silently.

The thought that one of them might not make it to see the next sunrise does not even cross my mind. It seems so far from possible. Hell, we had made it through some tough days already, why would today be any different?

The convoy rolls out of the gate like it has so many other times before. Today we roll with a few extra assets: tanks, Bradley fighting vehicles, and one of our sister platoons. Boy, was it a sight to see! We all understand today is going to be a big deal.

None of us expects it to start so quickly. Everyone is scanning the rooftops as the convoy enters the city. We know this village and we know we are not welcome! That is why we are here. First enemy contact comes quickly…small arms fire from multiple targets. A loud explosion rocks the center of our convoy.

Was that an IED or an RPG? I wonder.

It is too soon to tell. The radios start chattering back and forth between convoy and command. It is all just noise. I can't make out the words. The vehicles keep rolling. The sounds of gunshots are ringing out all around us. They seem to be coming from every direction.

Now suppressing fire from our convoy is making it even more chaotic. The wretched stench of gunpowder is filling the air. A smell so thick it is burning our lungs. Smoke is covering the roadway; we push through! I fire blindly into the darkness, hoping my rounds are finding an enemy target…a target that I can't see.

"Hell, this is not what I expected when the mission began early this morning," I say to myself.

The adrenaline's flowing strong now! Everything seems to move in slow motion. It's like something out of a movie. I experienced this same feeling in April of that year. That feeling of uncontrolled chaos returns. The truth is, I kind of liked it. I think that when death is an option, life just feels more real. In that moment, every detail is crisp. Over the years, I still get that feeling sometimes. Even as I write this now, I can feel my heart race, just a little.

We arrive at the Agricultural Building just as the sun starts to break the horizon. As the sun's rays beam through the smoke, it makes it even more difficult to see. The building is huge compared to others in the area. It is three stories high.

This could work. We can hold this position, I think to myself. *The plan is to stop chasing the enemy and make them come to us.*

This building in the heart of the city should do it. As we pull in, everything goes silent. An ominous silence for the moment, as the gunshots stop. As we begin to set up our stronghold everyone is moving a little faster today. Vehicles are positioning in the courtyard. Weapons are training on the houses surrounding us. The wall is only five feet high. The tops of the vehicles clearly concern me. Brave men slide up through the gunners' hatches and begin scanning the buildings around us.

Those houses—those civilian houses. Civilian houses that hide an enemy from our view, my thoughts speak loudly to me!

We know that today will yield death and destruction for this village.

This is a strange feeling to know death is riding with you for the day. There is no feeling of empathy for our enemy. We have had enough. We want to send a message! By next sunrise, that message will be loud and clear.

I take the time that morning to set up a casualty collection point just like I had so many times before. I search out an interior room with no windows, and away from where I thought the highest likelihood of damage might be sustained. I double check; triple check all my equipment. I foolishly think I will have enough for the day. I am quickly proven wrong.

Now a shot here, a shot there. A sniper lurking amongst the buildings surrounding us. Taking his shots when he can. A silent enemy until the shot rings out. It sounds like a crack of a whip. I HATE that sound. I can still hear that sound today. The men on the top of buildings crawling through the melting tar that coats the roofs stay low as sniper shots zip by just over their heads. They break out pieces of an already short wall to get their weapons in place—leaving themselves exposed.

I see them throughout the day. Their uniforms covered in that sticky substance. More small-arms fire coming. A few RPGs. This continues through the morning. It seems like this day will be like others before it. It has yet to show us what it truly held for us. The heat is overwhelming. I do not think I have ever experienced another day as hot as this. The hot Iraqi sun is baking. *It feels like we are on the surface of the sun!*

Sweat is pouring down from my forehead and quickly drying on my face. One by one, Soldiers rotate into the makeshift aid station I have set up. I spend my day dumping IV fluids into them to keep them in the fight.

The IV bags hung from the walls, discarded IV needles placed in one of the many empty water bottles that are littering the floor of the room. I started with over 100 IVs that day. *When the resupply came, I never thought I would be so happy to see a box of IV fluids.*

In an instant, everything changes!

We had been fighting an enemy that was spread throughout the town. We had caught them off guard with our early arrival. Now, our enemy has organized…this is THEIR city. They have positioned themselves all around us. Mortar fire is walking in on our position. It gets closer and closer. The *whoosh* of an RPG is heard, never making the contact it was meant for.

Our own artillery is almost melodic as it finds its target in the palm groves to the rear of our position. The tanks and Bradleys move through the streets around us, clearing what they can of our enemy. With all we had done up to this point, we have never experienced combat at this level.

WHY MY HEART IS PURPLE

This was it. This is what we had all been trained for. But no amount of training could prepare us for what happens next. The crack of a single round rings out. Quickly followed by a barrage of outgoing fire. The .50 cal sings out.

Now I believe there are only a handful of moments in life that define a person. For me, this was one of those moments. It was in this moment I realize what truly it meant to be called "DOC." A name given so quickly by these men who trusted me with their lives. The screams for a medic echo in my head. So much fear in that moment. There is no time to indulge it. Without a second thought, bag in hand, out the door I go.

The heat, the dry Iraqi heat beats down hard on my neck. The glare from the sun fills my eyes. It is almost disorienting. A light cloud of smoke still rolls from the top of the gunner's hatch. There I see him being lowered from the vehicle by his brothers. It is James!

Not 15 minutes before, I had seen him in the stairway smiling. I had told him to move…that where he was sitting was not safe. Like anywhere in that building was safe. The entire country was unsafe. That is the true irony of my job. I am to keep Soldiers safe in the middle of a war zone. It is an impossible task.

Now his body seems limp as he is placed on the ground. Frantically, I tear open his vest. I cut through the shirt, hoping to find some evidence of a wound. Again the .50 cal sing out! Hot brass pours from the top of the vehicle like a waterfall. I grab them as they fall on him.

My hands burning, I grip the spent shells. The sting of my own flesh being burnt just furthers my adrenaline high. I keep looking, looking for that wound. Blood on my hands tells me I have found it. My heart sinks.

We carry him inside. Our hands moving in a flawless symphony of medical care and treatment. I stop. He looks right at me. Not with the smiling face from before, but a face filled with fear.

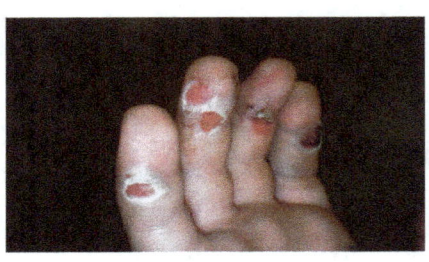

Sims' Burned Hand

I tell him, "It will be alright."

I lied. I did not know that my words would hold no truth. But maybe, in that moment, they brought some form of peace and comfort. We do what we can. We pray it is enough.

We move him to a nearby Bradley and load him up. We must get him to the evacuation point. We have to get him out of this damn village. The vehicle stops and the rear door begins to open. That sunlight is once again blinding us. The familiar sound of gunfire rings out again. A *whoosh* and another explosion. It is RPG fire, directed at us. A cloud of smoke and dust moves across the road where we stand as I look at the evac team. I know their faces. It is SGT. Blink.

Seeing him brought me a moment of peace. I yell, "Keep moving!"

I want to ignore the gunfire. It is like all the noise, all the smoke, and all the chaos disappears for just a moment. This will not be the last time I see their faces in this kind of situation. We pass him off to those medics, who do their best as well. And then we load up for our return into the frenzy.

I am dropped off 100 meters from the safety of the building. The blood rushing through my veins is pouring adrenalin into my heart once again. I and another Soldier run through the streets. Gunfire rings out, those horrible, hellish sounds filling our ears as we wait for the bullet to hit its mark. We know who the targets are. It is us. I can hear the bullets zipping by. Hitting the mud walls behind us. Neither of us is hit. So again, we sprint through the open, that 100 meters seemed like 100 miles as we run into the courtyard of the Agricultural Building. Suppressing outgoing fire flies over our heads, as we keep bolting all the way into the building.

I pause to catch my breath. Then walk down the long hallway. There, all those faces in the hallway are staring at me. Looking for some response or sign from me that their brother is okay. I have nothing for them. No comfort to offer. I step into the dark bathroom. I need a minute to compose myself. I pour a bottle of water down my back; I finally feel like I had composed myself enough to where they would not see my fear when I walk back out to face them. Maybe I did, maybe I did not.

I returned to finish the day of shooting and explosions. Mortars, RPGs, small arms and more sniper fire that no doubt found its target in James. My medic skills blossomed, and I found a love for what I do that day. Alongside some of the best medics I have ever served with, we kept our Soldiers in the fight. As I sit in my makeshift aid station that night, you can see that is what we have done. Under the glow of chem lights you could see the discharged bags of IV fluids we used to fight the overwhelming dehydration suffered by most that day. Blood stained the floor from where others had been treated for their wounds. The flow of Soldiers did not stop. Even in the early hours of the next morning, I found myself providing care to those who had given everything they had.

It is a day I cannot forget. A day where we saw death many times on both sides. A day where we watched as others were injured, but not nearly as grave as James.

In the back of my mind though, the question lingers, *Was he okay? Did he make it?*

We have not been told anything and I was afraid to ask even though I would not admit it at the time. So, we just pushed through. That day was hell for sure. I never experienced another quite like it. Or maybe others like it no longer carry that same weight. Maybe that day left me a different man. Numb to the chaos. Maybe, I still find myself looking back to that day. Fifteen years and it feels like yesterday.

As we came back to the safety of where we called home, we gathered once again. Twenty-four hours had passed since we stood there, saying the Lord's Prayer for safekeeping. This time, the faces around me look different. They are tired and weathered. No locker room enthusiasm as the words come out of the Lieutenant's mouth. The words I had been dreading all night. The words I hoped he would not say.

James had not survived his wounds. His wound, ever be it so small, had taken his life. No amount of battlefield care could have changed that. I know that now. But in that moment, I do not think there is even a word to describe how I felt. I felt the emotions rush over me. My Soldiers around me with tears in their eyes. I foolishly walk away. I walk out into the still dark morning and find a place where no one can see me. Then I wept, I cried like I had never cried before. I did not want them to see me. I wanted them to think DOC was strong. That I had it together. I wanted them to feel safe with me at their side, because tomorrow, we would again have to roll out those gates.

I was not alone! One of my Soldiers found me there. A crumbled mess is what I must have looked like. He gave me comfort.

I thought, *It's not supposed to work like this. I am supposed to be there for him.*

It's taken a long time for me to realize that sometimes, you must let someone else hold you up when you cannot do it yourself.

Not a day passes that I do not reflect on that 24 hours. I run through every moment searching for an explanation of why a young life was taken. He was still one of my Soldiers. My responsibility, my brother. I will never forget. That moment in time made me the medic and the man I am today. Rest in Peace Soldier. Your fight is done!

CHAPTER 4

TO HURT OR TO HEAL

First the Army taught me to kill and then they taught me to heal. This is a dilemma that many Combat Medics face in war. When to save a life and when to take a life? This is a hard question to ask yourself. This is a question that I have asked myself many times, and the answer is never easy. These stories tell of those times.

August 2005: A Soldier and a friend lay in the sand, blood pooling beneath his head. His lungs trying to breathe. His eyes fixed on nothing, head tilted to one side, legs and arms motionless. He is a young Soldier, maybe in his early twenties, a young man like any other, who should be in his freshman year in college or maybe looking for a summer job.

I think in my mind, *In less than five minutes he will most likely die, right here in the dirt of this horrible country. He will die in my arms. I will carry his blood stains on my boots and on the sleeves of my uniform.*

I possess the medical skills to save his life and my training as a war fighter helps me to think on my feet. I respond confidently, even brazenly, yet I understand that saving a patient with a head injury involves a lot of luck. Maybe this is one of those lucky days and my patient survives. I feel good. But I also feel that this Soldier with a shrapnel hole in his skull, might eventually wish I had let him die, in the sand thousands of miles from home with other Soldiers looking on.

But that is not my decision to make. I am here to save lives no matter what. My gut tells me this one particular patient has a chance to survive. It also tells me, if he ever makes it home, he will live in pain for the rest of his life.

Then it happens. The sound of another explosion and then small-arms fire. As I treat this Soldier the bullets are hitting the rock wall of the building we are hiding in. Now the decision to shoot back or to continue treating. Do I have to take a life to save a life? I know how to kill, but I do not want to. Taking a life is never easy even when it is the enemy. It is natural and unnatural, that genetic code, to know as much about killing as healing, to listen to the sounds of bullets in one moment, then listen for the sounds of the wounded in the next. Pull the trigger or pack the wound? First one then the other, the necessity of war.

That instant crossing from medic to Soldier and Soldier to medic without focusing on the difference between the two because in the end all that matters is just one thing—breathe like a Soldier in one breath, then breathe like a medic in the next.

The sounds of war, those chilling sounds. Fear makes its own kind of sound. Listen for the patterns, the ones that whisper about going home without legs or arms and the ones that mourn the painful deaths of fellow Soldiers. Learn to live with those deafening sounds, especially the ones telling you your medical skills may never be enough; that because of you a Soldier may live or die. Shake your fear and keep moving forward.

October 2005: A Soldier with a salvageable wound lies at my feet. Iraqi insurgents are attacking our position, and we need to clear the area fast. I stop to return fire. Even though I am trained to heal, I am also trained to kill, and that fact makes me a little hesitant. I laid that hesitation aside for just a moment and put on my warrior hat. Because after all we are at war. My gut tightens as I fire a round or two. I grab the Soldier by the collar of her uniform and jerk her torso up and off the sand, then sprint as fast as I can twenty yards.

As I run, the Soldier's legs drag and slow me down. Other Soldiers help me put her on a litter, so we can get the hell out of the kill zone. Her right leg dangles off to the side. A fellow medic grabs it and puts it back onto the litter. She screams so violently I can see the vessels in her neck distend and pulse. The leg is barely attached. It is covered with dirt and sand. The bones look like broken spears as they poke through her skin and the burned fabric of her uniform. She is losing blood faster than I know is sustainable for life, and I know if I do not get a tourniquet on her thigh right now—in the middle of this attack—she will bleed out and die. So I place the tourniquet and tighten it up. The tourniquet slips. Bones slice against her open wound. She starts bleeding again. Her leg is only attached by a few pieces of flesh and is causing more damage dangling there than it is doing good. I grab my trauma shears and detach the leg so I can reapply the tourniquet. I finally manage to get the tourniquet tightened again, and I am relieved I made the decision to remove the leg. We needed to move and dragging the leg was slowing everyone down, and the Soldier was better off alive, even without her leg.

Finally, the sound of helicopter rotor blades in the distance. I know they are coming to pick her up. I know I have done everything I can do to keep her alive, it is now up to the crew on the Blackhawk and the Trauma Team at the field hospital to do the rest. Later that night we received word that she had survived her wounds and would be on her way to the military hospital in Germany. We took pride in knowing we fought hard that day. Taking in the win knowing that tomorrow we may have to do it all over again.

As a medic, Soldiers will depend on you to make all the right decisions. I feel that all the right decisions are a blur, even though I have spent years in training just so my mind can never get blurred, so I can think without hesitation in the chaos and screaming of combat. I trained well, but I know all those war games and evac scenarios did not prepare me as much as I thought. How could they?

This is real. The fear and the blood and the shit are real. Death is real! War is real. And all I can do is adapt and breathe and try to hold on. So, I grasp my weapon and my ammo and my body armor. I carry them next to my medic bag, next to the bandages and tourniquets and the morphine. When I grab my gear, I never know what is going to happen. Despite what I feel, I move out anyway. As I do, I sense the mysterious alchemy of war has transformed me into something different, something stronger.

CHAPTER 5

OUR IRAQI BROTHERS

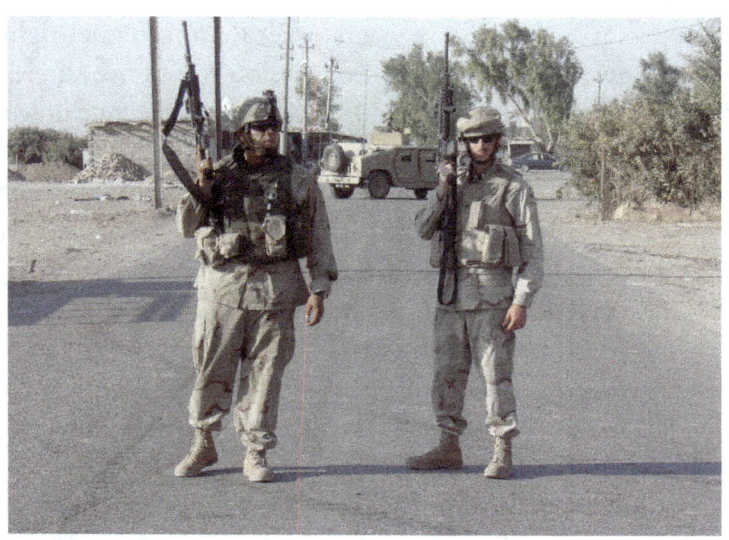

Sims with good friend Hererra on patrol in Baghdad.

When in war every day seems long. But some are longer than others, especially when you are a Combat Medic. The day was 7 March 2005, and it starts as most of my days start in Iraq—with a good Army meal and a prayer for protection. Today our team's mission was to do a presence patrol on the north end of Baghdad. This time we would be taking out our fellow Iraqi military partners that we had been working with and training for the past few months.

We had bonded with our Iraqi counterparts by this time and considered them brothers in arms. I had even been training one of them to be a medic. This thrilled me to pass on my skills and knowledge to an Iraqi who will take what he has learned to make his country a better place.

As the patrol rolls through the streets, streets that we had patrolled many times before, we feel a little more confident today. We have our Iraqi military friends with us, and we hope all would stay quiet, and it did for a while. Our patrol consists of 4 HMMWVs and the Iraqis have a flatbed pickup that they piled about 15 Soldiers into (not the safest thing to do).

As we continue down a very narrow alley it happens. A huge explosion, the biggest explosion I have ever seen in person, rocks the middle of the convoy. It has struck the Iraqi vehicle directly.

As smoke fills the air, I feel the concussion of the blast and my ears begin to ring. The Iraqi truck has driven directly over the IED as it detonated. The truck with 15 men rockets into the air. It has to be at least 15-20 feet. The vision of bodies flying everywhere still fills my memories to this day.

I am the only medic on the patrol today except for the Iraqi Soldier I had been training. As the smoke settled, I fear for him. I think there is no way any of them survived that blast. As the team secures the area all I want to do is get to those Iraqi Soldiers. I am desperate to see if I can help them. In times like this everything seems to slow down and waiting to get to them seems like it takes forever.

Finally, we are able to get to the blast sight. The first thing I notice is one of the Iraqi Soldiers pinned under the truck. When the vehicle landed after the blast, he was under it. I run to him, but it is already too late. I can tell he is dead. As I look around, I felt a rush of panic coming over me. There are bodies everywhere, and there is silence. Not one of them is making a sound. This tells me that none had survived the horrible fireball.

Then out of nowhere, a sound of hope, a sound of pain... *someone is alive.*

I move toward the moans and find him. The skin on his face is burned to the bone. It is like looking at a burned face of a skeleton. But he is still alive! I pause for a moment and start to tend to his burns. I scanned the rest of his body; his facial burns are his only injuries. I know he is in pain, hell, I am in pain just looking at him.

I gave him some morphine to ease his suffering, this is the least I can do. I reach for the back of his head to ensure he has no head wounds. As my hand brushes past his ear, to my horror it disintegrated like ashes blowing in the wind. I have never seen burned flesh do this. I wrap his face with bandages as best I can as screams and moans from others start to carry up into the air.

He is not the only survivor, there are others, my mind races.

Once again, I follow the muffled sounds and, in the wreckage, find two more men. The first man is up and walking around. Moving blindly. When he turns to face me, I realize his right arm is missing from the shoulder. Then he collapses. When I reach his position, I realize he also has a very severe abdominal wound. I take his pulse and do not feel a heartbeat.

Next to him is a pile of bodies, mostly unrecognizable body parts. A leg here and arm there. No amount of medical skills is going to save them now.

Are there anymore survivors? Was this it? my mind questions.

After scanning the entire area with my fellow platoon members, we determine that only one man has survived. Although he has survived the blast, would he survive his burns? Only time will tell. After securing the area and ensuring we could not save anyone else, we decided to take a small breather before moving on to the task we are all dreading.

We have to search for human remains and place them in body bags. As we drink cold water and have a few bites from an MRE, the smell of gunpowder, burned flesh and blood fills our noses.

All of us dread the task that lies before us. As we sift through the carnage of the blast site, we occasionally come across a foot, a toe, a leg, or arm. We try our best to respect these men and to handle their remains in a way we would want our bodies to be treated.

That evening back at the base we gather with more Iraqi Soldiers. Together we mourn the dead. They pray in their language, and we pray in ours; together we pray for those brave men to Rest in Peace for all eternity. We break bread together forging a bond of war that can never be broken, no matter what uniform you are wearing.

Chapter 6

BABY BOOM!

This story starts like many of the stories from my time in Iraq, with a briefing and a prayer before our team rolls out of the gates of Camp Taji, Iraq. Although it starts the same, it does not end in the way many of these stories end, with memories of gunfire and explosions.

This story ends with new life, instead of death and destruction. This is a story you would not expect to hear coming from a war zone.

The day was December 30th, 2015. Our team recently lost one of our brothers, James, in a firefight only 17 days prior. The pain of losing him was still fresh in our minds. Five days before this day was Christmas, but this was a Christmas like no other. We had recently lost a friend, a brother and teammate, so celebrating Christmas seemed to dishonor his name in some way.

Although we never mentioned it to each other I know we were all thinking it. Regardless, this Christmas we all sit around the tiny Christmas tree that someone received from a loving family member. We go to the dining facility for Christmas dinner, trying to keep our spirits up as best we can. We talk about James during dinner and decided we should call his wife to let her know we were thinking about her and James. That is a difficult but fulfilling phone call.

The call evokes a lot of tears, but I feel those tears are healing tears for her and for us. To be honest, after losing James we all wanted a little payback. But this day would not be about vengeance, revenge or hatred. Today it would be about a new life and new opportunity.

Our team has been given a mission of providing security for the Iraqi election. This was a mission we were not used to. Our missions typically called for seeking out and eliminating insurgents, so this is a new one for the team. Like every other mission before this one, I checked and double checked my gear, my weapon, and my medical supplies, because although we were not looking for a fight today the enemy may be looking for one. I was not about to lose another friend if I could help it. My job for today was the same as every day, provide medical support for my team. I had their backs and they had mine.

We arrived at the election site and set up a perimeter to secure the area the best we could. I set up my makeshift aid station in the back of my 113-track ambulance, just like I had done 100 times before. I hoped for the best and prepared for the worst. As we got everything prepared for the day, I walk the perimeter to check on my fellow teammates, to see if anyone needs anything from me before the Iraqi voters start to arrive.

After doing my rounds and the giving of a few IVs, I decide to go back to my vehicle and check my equipment one more time. A few hours later the voters began to arrive (there were more than I expected) and there were a lot of women in the crowd. This is a significant day for Iraqi women. This is the first time that women are allowed to vote or to have a voice in their newly founded government. As they arrive everyone could see my little ambulance with the red cross, and as always many of them came to get what little medical treatment I can provide.

As the day goes on and it got hotter and hotter, more and more voters arrive. Having this many people in one area makes me nervous. All it would take is one guy with an AK47 or a bomb vest to take out hundreds in the growing crowd. The day moves forward slowly, but without incident, and then it happened!

I heard the words every Combat Medic both hates and loves to hear—MEDIC!!! ...We need a medic!"

We hate those words because we know someone is hurt; we love those words because we know we are there to help. I recognized the voice, it was Tim, one of my team members.

The first thing that enters my mind, *I am not ready for this again so soon*, but then it hit me. I did not hear a gunshot or an explosion, *Maybe this is not going to be as bad as I think*.

I followed the screams for a medic, fearing the worst. Finally, I find Tim. Next to Tim is a very pregnant Iraqi woman. She has shown up to cast her vote along with her husband. What happens next, I am not prepared for. The woman nine months pregnant is in labor. She is having this baby right here in the Iraqi sand. I grab my interpreter so that I could talk to the woman.

Through the translator she says, *"I am going to have this baby right now!"*

Now let me tell you, the Army taught me how to take a life, and then taught me how to save a life, but had never really taught me how to bring a new life into the world. Although delivering a baby was part of my medic training, it was not something the Army spent much time on during my 10 weeks of Combat Medic Training. Because let's be honest, how many medics are put in a situation to deliver a baby in a combat zone? Although I was not ready for the task that lay before me, I knew I was the only one there that had the knowledge or skill to do it (regardless of how little skill I had in the task).

I carry the woman to the back of my ambulance and look to see what I am working with. Let me tell you, I have seen some of the most gruesome combat injuries, from amputations to severe gunshot wounds. I thought I had seen it all and that I was prepared for anything.

None of those combat wounds could have prepared me for this. Looking at the business end of an Iraqi woman about to give birth was worse than any combat wound I had seen before or since. Maybe it was because I had become numb to seeing combat wounds, maybe it was because I was scared that I did not have the skill to deliver this baby. But looking directly at the task before me I felt my heart racing. I could already see the head, so I knew the moment was close.

As the interpreter translated, I tried to tell her to **"Breath!"** like in the movies.

Not really sure I knew what I was doing, I cleaned the area as best I could with sterile water, as the contractions started again. I told the interpreter to tell her to push, and she did. We went through this routine for about 45 minutes. Finally, there I was with a newborn

Iraqi baby in my hands. I clamped off the umbilical cord and cut it with my pocketknife (I cleaned it with alcohol first). I cleaned the little guy off with IV fluids and cleaned out his nose, mouth and ears with a syringe.

While doing this, he did not make a sound, so I was a little worried. I know from movies that you are supposed to slap a baby on the butt to make them breathe, but mom and dad were right there watching me. So, I was a little scared to just slap him. Before I could do anything…the dad slapped his new son right on the butt and he started to cry. I guess things are the same in Iraq as they are in America when it comes to slapping babies after they are born. I then handed the baby to the mom, and she looked so happy. After 30 minutes or so of laying in the back of my ambulance and feeding the baby, the mom says something to the interpreter.

The interpreter says, *"She wants to leave the baby with you, so she can get back in line to vote with her husband."*

So, there we are, a group of Soldiers with M-16s holding a newborn Iraqi baby that I just helped deliver in the middle of a combat zone. The woman and her husband get back in line and cast their vote. While they are gone, I could not take my eyes off that little guy. I held him close because I was not about to let anything happen to him. I would protect him with my life, if necessary, as would have anyone on my team.

When they returned, the family asked my name and then I asked for theirs. They thanked me and I gave them the American flag patch from my uniform. Unfortunately, I never got to see them again. Who knows, maybe there is a 15-year-old Iraqi boy out there named Matthew!

That night at Camp Taji, we sat around the MWR facility talking and joking about the day's events. After thinking about it for a while I realize what a powerful day it has been. This day was better than most, because instead of taking a life we were able to bring a new life into the world. If you really think about it, this is a powerful story that showed some Iraqi people were ready for democracy. Not only was a baby born on this day, but democracy was also born for this family. It was so important for this woman to vote that she left her newborn child with a group of complete strangers with guns. This Iraqi family will never forget the day an American Soldier delivered their firstborn son. *War is hell but this day was a blessing from Heaven.*

Chapter 7

DOVE FOR DINNER

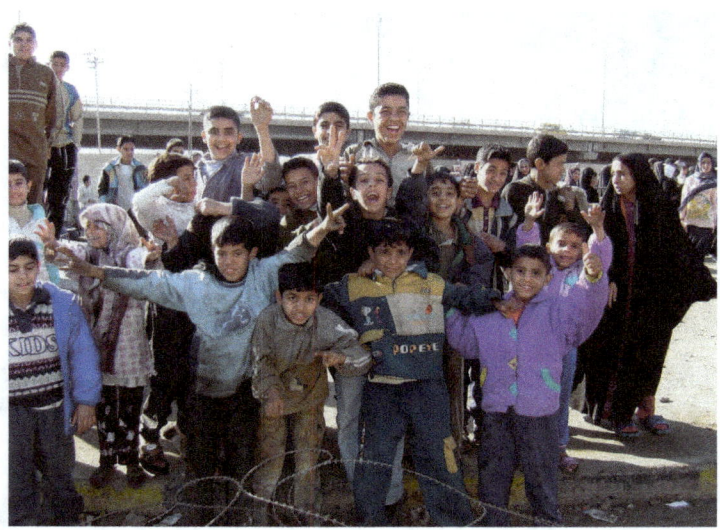

Iraqi children always came out to greet us when we were on patrol. We gave them the American candy and toys they loved.

Soldiers build bonds in war. That bond is not just between them, but also between the citizens of the country they are fighting in. As we patrolled the streets of Iraq, we relied heavily on the Iraqi citizens to help us weed out insurgents. But to do this we had to build bonds with them, we had to win their hearts and minds.

There was a particular family that I really enjoyed talking to. We visited them often and always had positive communication. The family consisted of the husband, wife, and a small 7-year-old boy. The husband even spoke a little English. When we would stop by randomly, they would always go out of their way to make us feel welcome. They would prepare tea for us and occasionally they would allow us to break bread with them.

This went on for months. The husband would keep us informed of any insurgent activity that was happening, and in return we would provide them with food and water. One of my favorite things to do was to bring candy to the little boy. Candy is not very common in Iraq, especially American candy. The smile on his face was always so big when he would see us coming. He knew his sweet tooth was about to be tickled soon.

Often, I would sit with him. He would teach me some Arabic and I would teach him a few words in English. No bad words. I promise. Well, maybe a few bad words. One day I asked his father when his son's birthday was. For the life of me I cannot remember what that day was. I also asked him what his son wanted for his birthday.

He said, "A soccer ball would be the best gift he could get. The ball he has is very old and will not hold air anymore."

So that night I went to the small military exchange on base and bought three soccer balls. One bright red, one bright blue and the other white. I wanted the balls to be something special. I wanted them to make a statement. What makes a better American statement than RED, WHITE, and BLUE?

His birthday was still three weeks away. I could hardly wait to give these soccer balls to this little Iraqi boy. Finally, the day came. It was time to have a birthday party. That day I bought some Twinkies at the PX. They were going to be his birthday cake.

We arrived at the house and there he was. He looked happy to see us.

"Happy birthday. I have something special for you," I said opening my bag and those soccer balls started bouncing on the floor.

He said in perfect English, "Those for me?"

When I shook my head, yes, he ran around the house screaming something. To this day I do not know what he was saying, but they seemed like happy screams. I played with him for about 15 minutes and then it was time for the Twinkies. I have never seen a kid look at Twinkies like this boy was looking at them. His intent glare said, "Twinkies, you don't stand a chance." In one minute, they were gone.

His father thanked us for what we had done and offered us to stay for dinner. We declined, because we had to be on our way. On the way out, I noticed that there were two doves in a cage, which I had not seen before.

I asked, "When did you get these?"

"They are my son's birthday gift," he answered.

As we were leaving, I told the father they are nice birds and that in America some people eat doves. Not giving it a second thought we said our goodbyes and headed back to base.

I few weeks later we had coordinated with the father to talk to him about the possibility of a local insurgent group in the area. When we arrived, I smelled something cooking. It smelled really good. I guess anything smells good after eating Army chow for months at a time. What I did not notice when we first arrived was there were no doves in the cage. Eventually they invited us to dinner, and I asked what we were having. The father pointed at the dove cage and said something in Arabic. Then it dawned on me. We are having his son's birthday doves for dinner.

I was dumbfounded and did not know what to say. I guess when I told him some Americans eat doves, it got lost in translation, and he thought I said I wanted to eat the doves. Now I felt bad, but the deed had already been done.

So, I thought to myself, *What the hell. Bring on the doves.*

We sat around on the floor eating flat bread, dove and drinking tea, while the little boy played with his soccer balls. It did not seem like he missed his doves at all. That was the best and only dove I have ever eaten.

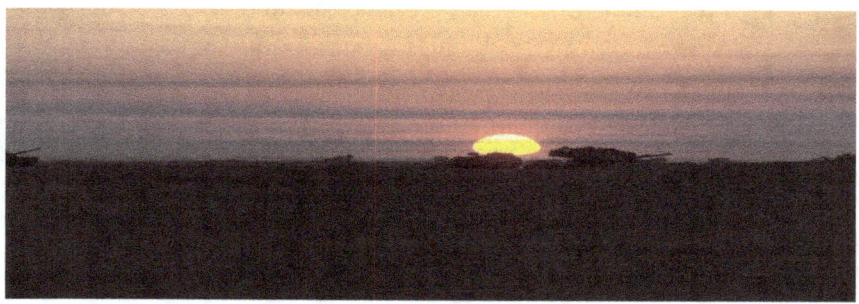

Chapter 8

RIGHT PLACE RIGHT TIME TO SAVE A LIFE

As a Combat Medic you are expected to save lives on the battlefield. I have used my medical skills many times while at war. But those skills have also been put to the test off the battlefield. It seems I find myself at the right place at the right time when help is needed.

April 2003: I was stationed in Germany. This particular day I was driving from Bamberg, Germany (where I was stationed) to Wuerzburg, Germany, to do Medical Proficiency Training at the military hospital in Wuerzburg. I was traveling on the Autobahn when I noticed a car was driving the opposite direction, against traffic (in Germany they call it a Ghost Driver).

Cars were swerving to avoid a head-on collision. I slowed down, but before I could fully stop a car in front of me could not get out of the way fast enough and was struck by the oncoming vehicle head on. I heard the sound of crumpling metal as pieces of both cars exploded into the air. I pulled over as other cars on the road were dodging the wreckage.

Finally, most of the vehicles came to a stop. My medic instinct kicked in and I moved towards the first car (the car that was driving against traffic). The occupants of the vehicle must not have been wearing their seatbelts. There were four passengers in that vehicle. Two of them had been ejected through the windshield and the other two were still in the car. Immediately I knew all of them were dead. I checked their pulse just to make sure. My instincts were correct. I moved to the other car that was involved.

There were two elderly passengers in this vehicle. Luckily, they were wearing their seatbelts. The elderly man was behind the wheel and his wife was in the passenger seat. The airbags had deployed, but both of them were unconscious. I checked their pulse, and they were both still alive.

One of the other Germans who had stopped called the German emergency services. I knew it was dangerous to move them, but I also knew it was dangerous to leave them there. I made the decision to move them to safety, away from the speeding traffic.

First, I lifted the man from the vehicle and moved him to the shoulder of the road. Going back for his wife, I realized the car was now on fire. Smoke was starting to fill the car and I could see flames coming from the hood. Soon they would spread to the cabin.

As I tried to lift the woman out, she would not budge. Her legs were pinned under the crumpled dashboard. I could feel the heat from the flames getting hotter and hotter and knew the time to save this woman was getting shorter and shorter. I tried desperately to free her legs, but they remained pinned.

My skin was starting to burn, and then it happened. There was a small explosion, and I was blown back about ten feet. My arm was on fire now as I slapped at the flames to put them out. Time was growing short as the flames grew higher and higher. I moved towards the car again to make one last effort to get this woman out of harm's way. I pulled hard and she slipped out. I guess the explosion had freed her legs.

Now she is awake! As I move her next to her husband and lay her down, I look back at the car and it is completely engulfed in flames. We both narrowly escaped being burned to death. Finally, the German ambulance service arrives and loads husband and wife into two separate ambulances. A few weeks later I was notified by the German police that they both survived.

Chapter 9

SOLDIER'S MEDAL

For my actions that day I was awarded the Soldier's Medal.

"The Soldier's Medal is awarded to any person of the Armed Forces of the United States who while serving in any capacity with the Army of the United States not serving in a duty status at the time of the heroic act, distinguished himself or herself by heroism not involving conflict with the enemy.

"The heroic act must have involved personal hazard or danger and voluntary risk of life under conditions not involving conflict with an armed enemy. It is the highest honor a Soldier can receive for an act of valor in a non-combat situation, held to be equal to or greater than the level which would have justified an award of the Distinguished Flying Cross had the act occurred in combat."

May 2018: Aboard the *Showboat Branson Belle*, my wife and I are enjoying a little time off in Branson, Missouri. That evening we decided to get tickets for the Showboat dinner cruise. It was going to be a special night. We do not get dressed up often, but tonight I was wearing my military dress uniform. The show starts and dinner has just been served. It is a packed show, and everyone is enjoying the music. As I eat my food and my foot was tapping to the music, I notice a woman in the front row stands up very quickly.

Now my many years as a Combat Medic have made it easy for me to spot when something is not right. Just the way she stood up seemed off to me. My instincts are right. She starts to grab at her throat, and immediately I know she is choking. Her husband gets behind her and starts to do the Heimlich maneuver (abdominal thrusts). As I moved towards them the show still going on, I could see the panic in their eyes. The abdominal thrusts were not working. As I approached, I told the husband I was a paramedic and that I was going to help. I began to do abdominal thrusts on the woman. It was not working; the food was not coming out. She was choking to death.

She started to turn blue and pass out. I knew that if I could not get this piece of food out, she was not going to make it. As I thought what do, it dawned on me. I can do a cricothyroidotomy to bypass the obstruction. But this was not a great environment to do this type of procedure. It involves cutting a hole in her neck and placing a tube for her to breathe through. But what choice do I have? I grab a steak knife and a plastic straw from the table.

At this point she is still conscious but is laying down on her back. As I prepared to make the cut in her neck, something tells me to try to do abdominal thrusts while she is laying down. I push on her abdomen very hard a few more times, and plop, the piece of chicken comes flying out. She took her first deep breath of air in approximately five minutes.

I tell her everything is going to be alight and to just relax and not to move. I monitored her for 15 minutes and then she says she wanted to get up. Her husband and I help her up and take her outside on the deck of the boat to get some fresh air. Eventually she said she was okay and wanted to get back to the show. The couple moved back to their front-row seats and the show never skipped a beat.

Later that evening they approached me and thanked me for helping them. The husband explained that he was in the military many years ago and asked where I was stationed. I told him Fort Sill and he said he was stationed there himself at one point of his career. The show ended and as we are leaving the woman once again thanks me for saving her life and gives me a hug.

After the weekend I returned to work at Fort Sill at the Reynolds Army Health Clinic. I was sitting in my office when I received an email from the Fort Sill Public Affairs Office. It seems that the husband had written an email to the Fort Sill Post Commander about what I had done, and they wanted to do a story for the local newspaper.

The husband wrote this email to the Commanding General of Fort Sill: "My wife and I were at the *Showboat Branson Belle* celebrating my retirement. During dinner, my wife got a piece of chicken lodged in her throat and was in a life-threatening situation. I was attempting the Heimlich maneuver unsuccessfully. Master Sergeant Sims moved me out of the way and said, 'I am an EMT' and took over. He was able to save my wife's life through his quick thinking and decisive manner."

CHAPTER 10

MAKING AN IMPACT

Military service brings people from all walks of life, all cultures, and many different beliefs together in one team. During my service I have been impacted by many people. These include the great leaders who built me into the leader I am today. Each man and woman I served with has touched my life in one way or another. One thing I never really gave much thought to was how I may have impacted them as well. When I retired from military service in 2019, I started to receive letters from Soldiers I had served with. These letters were more meaningful than any medal the Army could give me.

LETTER 1

My name is Mike and I hope it is okay that I am contacting you today. I served with Master Sergeant Sims in Iraq. I have been seeing a lot about him on Facebook, and was at the Memorial Day ceremony on Monday, and got to hear his speech. Someone gave me your information so that I could contact you. There is a lot more that Sims has done in his career, and I thought you would like to know more about him. I have also attached letters from people he has served with and others he saved. I plan to give these letters to him as soon as I get them all. See the story below. I am trying to make him famous because his story has the potential to motivate and make people take positive action.

Back in 2005 during the Iraqi elections the platoon that Sims and I were in was tasked with pulling security for one of the election sites. There were a lot of Iraqis that showed up at this voting site and the line was huge. Of course, it was a miserably hot day, standing around in the sun, but these Iraqis showed up to cast their vote. There were a lot of women there also. It was the first time they were allowed to vote. Sergeant Sims was our medical coverage that day, like every day. We were all standing by our tank eating MREs when we heard someone yelling for the Americans. An Iraqi man brought his wife over, and she was very pregnant and was going into labor. The entire family was there to vote that day. Sims did not even hesitate; he laid the woman down and then went and got the translator. What I witnessed after that was amazing. Sims delivered that baby right there. It was like he did it a thousand times before. After about an hour of making sure the baby and woman were okay the woman asked if she could go vote. It amazed me that this woman in the middle of a war zone would leave her baby with us. So, there he was taking care of a newborn Iraqi baby, carrying an M-16. While he was holding the baby, I will never forget what Sims said. He said this is why we are here. No matter if you support the war or not right here, what happened today makes it all worth it. All of the hot miserable days, being away from our family, all the friends we have lost, today's events make all of the sacrifice worth it. And when you think about it that is true. This Iraqi family has such a great picture of Americans in their mind. They will never forget the day an American Soldier helped bring their son into the world.

LETTER 2

To my favorite Medic in the world. On the occasion of your retirement after 22 years of service to our country. I want to remind you how many lives you have touched with your leadership and compassion. You sir have touched so many lives with your healing hands. Soldiers under your leadership have grown to be better Soldiers and have passed that legacy on to their Soldiers. When we served together in Iraq, I was always in awe watching you work. The platoon always felt safer with you there. What I remember most about you was that you were always the first to wake up and the last to go to bed each night. You would wake up before everyone else and load your backpack along with your aid bag. Your backpack was filled with everything to make a Soldier heal. You would walk the perimeter every morning to check on all of the guards in the towers. To see if they needed any medical care and you always had a snack or cold water to hand them. You did the same thing each evening before going to bed. You did all of this after going on every patrol. When the Soldiers were resting you were out making sure they were ready for the next day of patrols. You are a patriot, and this country is stronger because of your service. I wish you all the best in your retirement. Your eternal friend, Chad.

LETTER 3

Dear Mr. Sims, my name is Thomas, and you saved my son Larry's life in Iraq. I was told that you retired from service recently and I want to take this opportunity to thank you. Because of what you did for Larry I have been able to spend every Christmas with him for the past 14 years. He is alive today because of you and now has a wife and two children. I love my grandchildren. Without you they would not be in my life. I hope you continue to find happiness because you have made me the luckiest dad in the world. To my guardian angel, thank you, Thomas.

LETTER 4

Mr. Sims, although we have never spoken, we have met. Back in 2015 you saved my life on Interstate 40 in Arkansas. I wrecked my car and was pinned under my truck. I am sure you remember that night better than me. I do not remember much from that night but what I do remember is seeing you and you telling me that you were there to help. I do not know if it was because of my injuries or if God himself was using you as one of his angels that night. But I remember seeing a bright light behind you the entire time you were helping me. Like you were glowing. My family and I are so grateful that you were driving behind me that night. We can never repay you for what you did. All I can say is thank you. Sincerely, Walter R.

LETTER 5

To DOC Sims, I don't think I could ever express to you how grateful I am to have served with you. First and foremost, thank you for saving my life. You risked your life to save me, and I can never say thank you enough. I get to be a dad to my girls because of you. I get to be a husband because of you. I get to be a son to my parents because of you. I treasure each day. One thing I can promise is that I will pay it forward. God bless you; God bless America, HAWK 6D.

LETTER 6

Hello Battle Buddy, I cannot believe you actually gave up the uniform. I was sure you were going to be the Sergeant Major of the Army one day. In my eleven years of service, I have never seen a more dedicated medic & Soldier. No matter if we were deployed or back in Germany you seemed to never run out of energy. I was always amazed watching you work your magic medic hands. It was like God was using your hands as his tools. I hope that you find happiness in retirement and also find a way to continue to serve. Your Battle Buddy, Mike S.

LETTER 7

Hello Matt, wow it feels weird calling you Matt. I can't believe you actually retired. You were an awesome medic. This will sound crazy, but what I remember the most about you besides being a crazy medic is that you cured my horrible athlete's foot while we were in Iraq. I went to five doctors and was given so many meds, but nothing seemed to help, until you had me come in every day to soak my feet in peroxide, then put on the cream. My fungus was cured after two weeks and has never come back. Trust me, my wife loves you for that. Well, I hope you don't miss serving too much and good luck, Trevor W.

MY FAVORITE PATRIOTIC SPEECH

I want to end this section of the book by sharing an abridged excerpt of a speech from President Ronald Regan. The speech is called "A Soldier's Pledge."

"A SOLDIER'S PLEDGE" BY RONALD REGAN

If we look to the answer as to why for so many years we have achieved so much, prospered as no other people on Earth, it is because here in this land we unleashed the energy and individual genius of man to a greater extent that has ever been done before. Freedom and the dignity of the individual have been more available and assured here than in any other place on Earth. The price for that freedom at times has been high, but we have never been unwilling to pay that price. Those who say that we're in a time when there are no heroes, they just don't know where to look. The sloping hills of Arlington National Cemetery, with its row upon row of simple white marker bearing crosses or Stars of David. They add up to only a tiny fraction of the price that has been paid for our freedom. Each one of those markers is a monument to the kind of hero I spoke of earlier. Their lives ended in places called Belleau Wood, the Argon, Omaha Beach, Salerno, and halfway around the world on Guadalcanal, Tarawa, Pork Chop Hill, the Chosin Reservoir, and in a hundred rice paddies and jungle of a place called Vietnam. Under one such marker lies a young man, Martin Treptow, who left his job in a small-town barbershop in 1917 to go to France with the famed Rainbow Division. There on the western front, he was killed trying to carry a message between battalions under heavy artillery fire. We're told that on his body was found a diary. On the flyleaf under the heading, "My Pledge" he had written these words:

"America must win this war. Therefore, I will work, I will save, I will sacrifice, I will endure, I will fight cheerfully and do my utmost, as if the issue of the whole struggle depended on me alone." We must realize that no arsenal or no weapon in the arsenals of the world is so formidable as the will and moral courage of free men and women. It is a weapon our adversaries in today's world do not have. It is a weapon that we as Americans do have. Let that be understood by those who practice terrorism and prey upon their neighbors. As for the enemies of freedom, those who are potential adversaries, they will be reminded that peace is the highest aspiration of the American people. We will negotiate for it, sacrifice for it; we will not surrender for it now or ever.

The men and women portrayed in the pages of this book lend credence to the axiom that with diversity comes strength. They came from all walks of life and a wide variety of socioeconomic, ethnic, and racial backgrounds. They range from very young to late middle age. The fallen medical personnel were born and raised in all corners of our nation. Some came from the cities of the Northeast and Mid-Atlantic. Some hailed from the rural South. Others enlisted from the heartlands of the Midwest or the majestic Rocky Mountain region. Many were from the West Coast. A few came from other parts of the world to serve in the U.S. Armed Forces in hopes of achieving citizenship. Any of them could have been our next-door neighbor, but none of them could be called ordinary. Without exception, they distinguished themselves with great courage in the face of extraordinary danger and hardship.

SECTION 2

FOREWORD

This section is about a special group of Americans. The official term for what they do is front-line trauma care—which means their office is a battlefield—their job is to save others' lives while risking their own. The medical personnel profiled in this book all paid the ultimate price in the performance of their duty. They left behind devoted family members and friends who mourn, and a nation that will forever honor their deeds and memories. These fallen heroes were part of a profession requiring skill, compassion, and the kind of fortitude to be simultaneously a warrior and a healer. Their calling is all the more difficult on an unconventional battlefield against an enemy that targets civilians and does not recognize or obey the laws of war. Since September 11, 2001, the medical personnel of the U.S. military have met this challenge selflessly, and courageously. Amid the tragedies of war, these are some of the most poignant contemporary accounts to reach the American public: a Warrant Officer coming under attack to rescue an Iraqi child; a Sergeant drawing fire to allow his team to escape; a Corpsman racing into a battle to treat a wounded Marine; and many more. This book gives us 219 of these stories of sacrifice. Underlying all accounts is something Americans need to know—that altruism in war is not only possible, but a daily reality for the brave men and women of military medicine. These are the cries that few have ever heard, the calls that ring out when a Soldier, Marine, Sailor, or Airman is hit. Fewer still can know the split-second decisions these brave young men and women must make: Do they leave their protected position and scramble to the side of the casualty with rucksack, weapons, and other gear, or do they wait until the shelling or small-arms fire diminishes? How much time does the casualty have? How big of a risk is it to the medic and the casualty to scramble that 50 or so yards and carry him back, knowing full well that the enemy has little regard for the red cross on the sleeve? Some 30,000 times our Medics and Corpsmen have faced that decision in Iraq and Afghanistan—whether to stand when others are diving for cover. For 219 of them, it was the last decision they made.

THOSE WHO GAVE IT ALL

JEFFERSON D. DAVIS
Died: December 5, 2001
Branch: U.S. Army

Master Sergeant Jefferson Davis was killed on December 5, 2001, when a bomb dropped from a B-52 landed near his position north of Kandahar, Afghanistan. Two other Soldiers were also killed. The 39-year-old Green Beret was assigned to the 3rd Battalion, 5th Special Forces Group at Fort Campbell, Kentucky, in support of Operation Enduring Freedom. Nearly 1,000 family, friends and comrades said goodbye to their fallen hero at the Elizabethton High School Gym in Tennessee, on December 18, 2001, and he was buried with full military honors at Happy Valley Memorial Park.

A survival training course roused Davis' interest in the military, and he enlisted in the Army in August 1983. He served in Korea for three years as a medical specialist before graduating from Special Forces Qualification Course and receiving his assignment to the 5th Special Forces Group (Airborne) in Fort Campbell, Kentucky. He went on to serve as a medical sergeant on both Operational Detachments, and completed a tour as senior instructor at the Special Warfare Center at Fort Bragg, North Carolina.

He then returned to the 5th Group, where he was selected to be the team sergeant for Operational Detachment A 574. During his time in the military, Davis served in Operation Desert Storm and numerous contingency operations throughout Southwest Asia. He deployed on his final tour in October 2001.

MATTHEW J. BOURGEOIS
Died: March 27, 2002
Branch: U.S. Navy

U.S. Navy Chief Petty Officer Matthew J. Bourgeois, a Hospital Corpsman, was killed on March 27, 2002, when he was serving in Operation Enduring Freedom. His death resulted from wounds sustained when he stepped on a land mine while conducting small unit training at Tamak Farms, an abandoned al-Qaeda base near Kandahar, Afghanistan. The 35-year-old Navy SEAL was assigned to the Navy Special Warfare Development Group, Little Creek Naval Amphibious Base, Norfolk, Virginia. He had been serving in Afghanistan for approximately two months and was slated to return to the United States in another month. A memorial service was held at the base chapel of Little Creek Naval Amphibious Base in Norfolk, Virginia, on April 5, 2002. Bourgeois began his career in the Florida National Guard, serving with that component from 1984 to 1987. He subsequently enlisted in the Navy. He trained as a Hospital Corpsman and later underwent Navy SEAL training in San Diego. During his 14-year tenure as a SEAL, he deployed in support of the first Persian Gulf War and continued to serve honorably up to the time of his death.

Matthew left behind his beloved wife, Michelle; his son Matthew Jr.; and his parents, Tom and Mae.

JASON D. CUNNINGHAM
Died: March 4, 2002
Branch: U.S. Air Force

Senior Airman Jason Dean Cunningham was killed in Afghanistan on March 4, 2002, in a rescue mission in support of Operation Anaconda, during Operation Enduring Freedom. Cunningham died from injuries sustained from enemy fire while he was selflessly treating wounded comrades on a mountain ridgeline in enemy territory on the deadliest day of combat for an American unit since 1993. He was laid to rest at Arlington National Cemetery in Arlington, Virginia. The ceremony included full military honors, a flyover by a pair of HH-60G Pave Hawk helicopters, and a 21-gun salute. A final heartbreaking salute was made by Jason's four-year-old daughter, Kayla, as her father was laid to rest in an American flag draped casket.

Jason's military career began in February 1995 when he enlisted in the Navy. Although he had once wanted to be a search and rescue swimmer for the Navy and had already passed the fitness test for the Navy SEALS, he instead decided to train to become an Air Force Pararescueman. He left the Navy and joined the Air Force in 1999 to fulfill his dream of becoming a pararescueman. He completed his 21-month Pararescue training in June 2001.

Jason is survived by his wife, Theresa, and their two daughters, Kayla and Hannah. He is also survived by his parents, Lawrence and Jackie Cunningham, his sister, Lori, and his brother, Chris.

JERRY O. POPE, II
Died: October 15, 2002
Branch: U.S. Navy

Ensign Jerry O. Pope, II, a 35-year-old Navy SEAL, was killed on October 15, 2002, in a traffic accident in Yemen while serving his country in support of Operation Enduring Freedom. Pope was assigned to the Intelligence Department at the American Embassy in Yemen and was participating in a training exercise with the Yemeni Special Forces. Family and friends celebrated his life on October 21, 2002, at the Naval Amphibious Base, Little Creek Chapel in Norfolk, Virginia, and again on October 30 at Marine Corps Base Quantico Chapel in Quantico, Virginia. He was buried at Arlington National Cemetery on November 21, 2002, where family, friends, and teammates said their final farewells to their fallen hero.

Jerry leaves behind his wife, Andrea; and young children Drew, Leah, and Jack.

CHRISTOPHER J. SPEER
Died: August 6, 2002
Branch: U.S. Army

Sergeant First Class Christopher J. Speer, an Army Special Forces Medic attached to the U.S. Army Special Operations Command, Fort Bragg, North Carolina, died on August 6, 2002, from injuries sustained on July 27, 2002. He and four other Soldiers were wounded when their reconnaissance patrol was ambushed near Khowst in eastern Afghanistan. Speer was evacuated by air first to Bagram Air Force Base, then to Ramstein Air Base in Germany for evaluation and treatment. His wife flew to be with him for the last week of his life, and she made the decision to remove him from life support and donate his organs for transplant. His funeral was held on August 13, 2002, at Village Chapel in Pinehurst, North Carolina.

Christopher leaves behind his wife, Tabitha; his two children, Taryn and Tanner; and his brother, Todd.

PETER P. TYCZ, II
Died: June 12, 2002
Branch: U.S. Army

Master Sergeant Peter P. Tycz, II, died on June 12, 2002, in the crash of an Air Force MC-130H Combat Talon II aircraft, in Paktika Province, Afghanistan. The plane crashed after taking off from an airfield southwest of Gardez in rocky terrain near Bande Sardeh Dam. Tycz was a senior medic aboard the aircraft. At the time of his death, he was serving with the 3rd Special Forces Group out of Fort Bragg, North Carolina. His family held visitation at the Hamp Funeral Home on June 14, 2002.

Peter is survived by his wife, Tami; his five daughters, Felicia, Faith, Tiffany, Samantha, and Elizabeth; his parents Peter and Paula; and his sister, Tracy.

MICHAEL C. BARRY
Died: February 1, 2003
Branch: U.S. Army

Sergeant Michael C. Barry, an Army Medic, died in an accident in Doha, Qatar, on February 1, 2003. In support of Operation Iraqi Freedom, he was a member of the 205th Area Support Medical Battalion, Missouri National Guard, Kansas City. Barry was buried with military honors on February 11, 2003, at the Shawnee Mission

Memorial Gardens, Lenexa, Kansas.

Michael is survived by his wife, Jennifer; and his parents, Michael and Maria Barry.

WILLIAM M. BENNETT
Died: September 12, 2003
Branch: U.S. Army

Sergeant First Class William M. Bennett, an experienced Soldier and Medic, was killed in the line of duty in the early hours of September 12, 2003, outside the town of Ar Ramadi, Iraq, in support of Operation Iraqi Freedom. Bennett served in the Army for 17 years and was most recently assigned to the 3rd Battalion, 5th Special Forces Group. His unit was carrying out a raid on enemy forces in a villa outside Ar Ramadi when a firefight erupted. The battle took the lives of Bennett and Master Sergeant Kevin N. Morehead of Little Rock, Arkansas, and wounded seven other men. His funeral was held on September 20, 2003, at Oak View Baptist Church in Walland, Tennessee, and he was buried in Oak View Cemetery in Walland.

Bill is survived by his wife, Allison, and son, Seth, as well as his parents, Leonard and Kathleen Bennett.

RICHARD P. CARL
Died: May 9, 2003
Branch: U.S. Army

Sergeant Richard P. Carl was killed on May 9, 2003, when the UH-60A helicopter on which he was flying as crew chief collided with a power line over the Tigris River, near Samarra, Iraq, during the rescue of a wounded Iraqi child. The crew was maneuvering to avoid enemy ground fire when the helicopter struck the wires. Carl was assigned to the 571st Medical Company, an air ambulance unit out of Fort Carson, Colorado. They were deployed to Iraq to support Operation Iraqi Freedom. Two pilots onboard were also killed, and a medic was rescued from the river in critical condition. Carl was buried in the

Glenn Rest Cemetery, Glenns Ferry, Idaho.

Carl was posthumously promoted to Sergeant. He is survived by his wife Audrey; his daughter, Early Ann, and his son, Dominick.

HANS N. GUKEISEN

Died: May 9, 2003
Branch: U.S. Army

Chief Warrant Officer Hans N. Gukeisen was killed on May 9, 2003, when the UH-60A helicopter that he was flying collided with a power line across the Tigris River near Samarra, Iraq. The crew had been dispatched to evacuate a wounded Iraqi child and was maneuvering to avoid enemy ground fire. Gukeisen was assigned to the 571st Medical Company. They were deployed to Iraq in support of Operation Iraqi Freedom. Two other crew members on board were also killed. Gukeisen was rescued from the river in critical condition, but later died of his wounds. He had been in Iraq for about six weeks when the accident occurred. His body was returned to Fort Carson for a unit memorial service at Butts Army Air Field. He is buried in Sturgis, South Dakota.

He is survived by his wife Holly; his parents Terry and Margaret; his grandmother, Eleanora; and his brother Raymond.

CHRISTOPHER J. HOLLAND

Died: December 17, 2003
Branch: U.S. Army

Specialist Christopher J. Holland, a 26-year-old Army medic, died December 17, 2003, in Baghdad, Iraq. While on patrol, his unit was ambushed and he was hit by small-arms fire as he tended to the wounds of his injured platoon leader. The courageous young Soldier was assigned to A Battery, 4th Battalion, 27th Field Artillery Regiment, 1st Armored Division and was garrisoned at Smith Barracks in Baumholder, Germany, supporting Operation Iraqi Freedom. Family and friends of the fallen hero gathered on December 23, 2003, to celebrate a pre-Christmas mass in honor of their beloved son at St.

Francis Xavier Catholic Church in Brunswick, Georgia. Holland was later buried in Arlington National Cemetery. Every Memorial Day without fail, Holland's family makes a trip to his gravesite, where they pray together as a family.

Specialist Holland was posthumously awarded the Bronze Star and the Purple Heart. Chris is survived by his parents, James and Mary Jo; and his sister, Amanda.

CRAIG S. IVORY
Died: August 17, 2003
Branch: U.S. Army

Specialist Craig S. Ivory, an Airborne Medical Specialist attached to the 501st Forward Support Company, 173rd Airborne Brigade, Southern Europe Task Force, Vincenza, Italy, died August 17, 2003, from a stroke after being in extreme battlefield conditions, including 135 degree heat while serving in support of Operation Iraqi Freedom. He was buried on August 23, 2003, with military honors, at the Indiantown Gap National Cemetery, Annville, Pennsylvania.

Craig is survived by his parents, Patrick and Terry; as well as his sister and two brothers.

MICHAEL MALTZ
Died: March 23, 2003
Branch: U.S. Army

Master Sergeant Michael Maltz, of the 38th Rescue Squadron, died on March 23, 2003, in Operation Enduring Freedom, when his HH-60 Pave Hawk Helicopter crashed in southeast Afghanistan. Maltz, along with five others on board, was on a humanitarian mission to provide medical evacuation for two seriously injured Afghan children. Master Sergeant Maltz was memorialized with a Mass of Christian Burial at St. Matthew Roman Catholic Church in Dix Hills, New York. He was buried with full military honors, including a gun salute and flyover by two military helicopters, at Pinelawn National Cemetery on Long Island. Maltz's family was presented with the flag that had been draped over the fallen hero's coffin.

Michael is survived by his sons, Kyle and Kody; his mother, Patricia; his father, John; his grandmother, Alice; his sister, Terri; and his brothers, Derek and Richard.

JOSHUA MCINTOSH
Died: June 26, 2003
Branch: U.S. Navy

Navy Hospital Corpsman Joshua McIntosh died on June 26, 2003, from injuries he received in a non-combat related shooting in Karbala, Iraq. The 22-year-old was assigned to the 3rd Battalion, 7th Marine Regiment, in Twentynine Palms, California, in support of Operation Iraqi Freedom. He was laid to rest in Willamette Memorial Park in Albany, Oregon.

Joshua is survived by his father, Dwaine McIntosh.

KEVIN N. MOREHEAD
Died: September 12, 2003
Branch: U.S. Army

Master Sergeant Kevin N. Morehead sacrificed his life for his country on September 12, 2003. His unit was conducting a pre-dawn raid on enemy forces in Ar Ramadi, Iraq, when he was struck by a bullet during the firefight. The 33-year-old Green Beret was assigned to the 3rd Battalion, 5th Special Forces Group in Fort Campbell, Kentucky. Master Sergeant Morehead was just two weeks shy of returning home, having volunteered to remain in Iraq to assist the replacement unit that had arrived to relieve his team. Friends and family gathered September 22, 2003, at Powell Funeral Home in Bald Knob, Arkansas, to celebrate Kevin's life. He was laid to rest with full military honors next to his grandfather in Fredonia Cemetery in Bald Knob.

Kevin is survived by his wife, Theresa; and his parents, Jim and Jeanette Morehead.

DAVID J. MORENO

Died: July 17, 2003
Branch: U.S. Navy

Petty Officer Third Class David J. Moreno, a 26-year-old Navy Hospital Corpsman assigned to the 4th Marine Division at Naval Medical Center, San Diego, California, lost his life July 7, 2003, from a non-hostile gunshot wound in Hamishiyah, Iraq. After completing a mission and unloading weapons, one of the guns accidentally discharged, killing Moreno instantly. Naval and Marine Reserve Units, including a color guard and rifle squad from Cheyenne, Wyoming, presented military honors during Moreno's funeral service.

David is survived by his parents David and Yolanda; and his two sisters, Holly and Sharlotte.

PAUL T. NAKAMURA

Died: June 19, 2003
Branch: U.S. Army

Specialist Paul T. Nakamura, an Army Reserve Soldier assigned to the 437th Medical Company, 3rd Medical Command Base in Colorado Springs, Colorado, was killed in action on June 19, 2003, on a highway in Iskandariyah, Iraq, 20 miles south of Baghdad. Supporting Operation Iraqi Freedom, Nakamura was part of a crew transporting an injured Soldier in the back of an ambulance when the vehicle was hit by a rocket propelled grenade that killed him and injured two other crewmen. On July 2, 2003, family, friends, and military personnel attended his funeral at Rose Hills Memorial Park in Whittier, California. He was the first Japanese American to be killed in the Iraq War.

In November 2003, the main living area of Convoy Support Center Scania was named Camp Nakamura in honor of Paul's memory.

JOSE AMANCIO PEREZ, III

Died: May 28, 2003
Branch: U.S. Army

Specialist Jose Amancio Perez, III, an Army Medical Specialist assigned to the 6th Battalion, 27th Field Artillery Regiment out of Fort Sill, Oklahoma, was killed in action on May 28, 2003, when the vehicle he was driving in Taji, Iraq, was ambushed and hit by a grenade. Although Perez was shot in the chest, he drove to a secure position, ensuring the safety of the three passengers in the HUMVEE. His courageous and heroic efforts epitomized his intense dedication to the welfare of those in his care. Emergency care failed to save his life, but his memory lives on.

On June 6, 2003, family, friends, and military comrades filled St. Francis de Paul Church in San Diego, Texas, for his funeral mass. He was buried in the San Diego City Cemetery with military honors.

Perez was posthumously awarded the Bronze Star and Purple Heart. He has been memorialized as one of 40 Texas Fallen Heroes, whose portraits were exhibited in a traveling display throughout the state of Texas in 2003. The display continues today with over 400 Texas sons and daughters who have lost their lives fighting the Global War on Terrorism.

JASON PLITE

Died: March 23, 2003
Branch: U.S. Air Force

Senior Airman Jason Plite died on March 23, 2003, near Ghazni, Afghanistan, while serving in support of Operation Enduring Freedom. A member of the 38th Rescue Squadron out of Moody Air Force Base, Georgia, Plite was killed when his HH060G Pave Hawk Helicopter crashed on its way to rescue two injured Afghan children. Funeral services for the fallen Airman were held at South Baptist Church near his family's home in Lansing, Michigan. Hundreds of mourners came to pay their respects. Following the service, Plite was buried at Delta Center Cemetery with full military honors, including a Color Guard and a 21-gun salute. A lone bugler played "Taps."

Jason is survived by his parents, Charlie and Dawn; siblings Alyssa and Shaynah.

TAMARRA RAMOS
Died: October 1, 2003
Branch: U.S. Army

SPC Tamarra J. Ramos, an Army Medic attached to the Medical Troop, Regimental Support Squadron, 3rd Armored Cavalry Regiment, out of Fort Carson, Colorado, died of cancer on October 1, 2003, at Walter Reed Army Medical Center. She had been evacuated from Iraq in August 2003 after she was diagnosed. Although she was treated with chemotherapy and other therapeutics, Ramos died at the medical center. Funeral services were held on October 9, 2003, at St. Paul's Evangelical Lutheran Church in Applebachsville, Pennsylvania.

Tammara is survived by her husband Eric; her parents David and Mary; her brother, David; and her sisters Melanie, Dia, Miriamani, and Kamaria.

JOHN R. TEAL
Died: October 23, 2003
Branch: U.S. Army

Captain John R. Teal lost his life on October 23, 2003, when an improvised explosive device exploded near his convoy near Baqubah, Iraq. The 31-year-old Medical Service Corps officer was assigned to Headquarters Company 2nd Brigade Combat Team, 4th Infantry Division in Fort Hood, Texas, supporting Operation Iraqi Freedom. Friends and family honored their son and brother on November 3, 2003, at St. Peter's United Methodist Church in Montpelier, Virginia, after which he was given a hero's burial on November 4, 2003, in Arlington National Cemetery, Arlington, Virginia.

John is survived by his parents, Joseph and Emmie; and his sister Elizabeth, as well as many extended family members and friends.

BRIAN K. VAN DUSEN

Died: May 9, 2003
Branch: U.S. Army

Chief Warrant Officer Brian K. Van Dusen was killed on May 9, 2003, when the UH-60A helicopter he was piloting as aircraft commander collided with a power line over the Tigris River. The crew had been dispatched to evacuate a wounded Iraqi child and was maneuvering to avoid enemy ground fire when they struck the wires. Van Dusen and aircraft were assigned to the 571st Medical Company based out of Fort Carson, Colorado. Two other crewmembers on board were also killed. A mass for the fallen hero was held May 19, 2003, at Holy Family Catholic Church in Security, Colorado.

Brian is survived by his wife Bridgette; children, Joshua, Kelly, Angel, and Joseph; parents, David and Jacqueline; and his sister Victoria.

MICHAEL VANN JOHNSON, JR.

Died: March 25, 2003
Branch: U.S. Navy

Petty Officer Second Class Michael Vann Johnson, Jr., of Little Rock, Arkansas, died in the line of duty on March 25, 2003. The 25-year-old Corpsman was assigned to the Naval Medical Center San Diego, 1st Marine Division Detachment, out of San Diego, California, in Support of Operation Iraqi Freedom. Johnson was killed by grenade shrapnel while riding in a HMMWV with the 3rd Battalion, 5th Marine Regiment, the unit he was assigned to care for in Iraq. Mourners filled the Agape Church in Little Rock, Arkansas, to pay tribute to the fallen hero on April 16, 2003. As fellow Sailors bade their final farewells with a 21-gun salute, Johnson was laid to rest at the Arkansas State Veterans Cemetery in North Little Rock.

Posthumously, Johnson was awarded the Purple Heart and promoted to Petty Officer Second Class. Michael is survived by his wife, Cherice; his father, Michael Sr.; his mother, Jana and seven siblings.

RONALD W. BAKER

Died: October 13, 2004
Branch: U.S. Army

Sergeant Ronald W. Baker died on October 13, 2004, of injuries sustained on October 7 when a vehicle borne IED detonated near his patrol vehicle in Taji, Iraq. Baker was a Medical Supply Specialist assigned to the 39th Support Battalion, Arkansas Army National Guard. He was buried with military honors at the Arkansas State Veterans Cemetery, in North Little Rock on October 21, 2004. To honor his memory, his hometown declared the day of his funeral "Sergeant Baker Day." He was promoted posthumously to Sergeant.

Ronald is survived by his wife, Joanne; and their daughter, Alexis.

PABLITO PENA BRIONES, JR.

Died: December 28, 2004
Branch: U.S. Navy

Hospital Corpsman Briones, Jr., died on December 28, 2004, while serving his country in support of Operation Iraqi Freedom. A native of Anaheim, California, the 22-year-old died as a result of a non-combat related incident in Fallujah, Iraq. His home unit was the 1st Marine Division Detachment, Naval Medical Center San Diego.

On January 3, 2005, California Governor Arnold Schwarzenegger ordered capital flags flown at half-staff in honor of Pablito. The governor said, "The loss of Seaman Briones is felt deeply by all who knew him. His memory will live on in his community, through his loved ones, those who served with him, and those who enjoy freedom because of his sacrifice."

DAVID A. CEDERGREN

Died: September 11, 2004
Branch: U.S. Navy

Petty Officer Third Class David A. Cedergren died accidentally from electrocution on September 11, 2004, in Iskandariyah, Iraq. He was assigned to the 2nd Marine Division, in support of Operation Iraqi Freedom. David was laid to rest at Fort Snelling National Cemetery in Minneapolis, Minnesota.

David is survived by his father and stepmother, Bart and Pam; his mother, Deb; two brothers, Barry and Brad; and two sisters, Jodi and Kristy.

RUSSELL L. COLLIER

Died: October 3, 2004
Branch: U.S. Army

Sergeant Russell L. Collier, an Army Medic, was killed on October 3, 2004, when, without thought for his own safety and carrying only his medic bag, he ran to the aid of Sergeant Christopher Potts, who had been hit by small-arms fire in Taji, Iraq. Collier had carefully disarmed himself so that he could quickly render aid to the injured Soldier. While he advanced under direct enemy fire, he was killed. Collier served with the 1st Battalion, 206th Field Artillery Regiment, 39th Infantry Brigade Arkansas National Guard, in support of Operation Iraqi Freedom. He was buried with military honors on October, 12, 2004, at Springfield National Cemetery in Springfield, Missouri.

For gallantry, Sergeant Collier was posthumously awarded the Silver Star, and during his dedicated service he received the Distinguished Service Medal, and Purple Heart.

Russell is survived by his wife, Rocky; his children, Hunter, Mary, Virginia, and Wayne; and his sister, Carolyn.

EDGAR P. DACLAN, JR.

Died: September 10, 2004
Branch: U.S. Army

Specialist Edgar P. Daclan an Army Medic attached to the 1st Battalion, 18th Infantry Regiment, 1st Infantry Division in Schweinfurt, Germany, was killed on September 10, 2004, when an improvised explosive device (IED) detonated near his patrol in the central Iraqi city of Baghdad. His unit had been responding to indirect fire from a covered position where the enemy could not be seen. He was leading the way when the homemade bomb exploded. He was buried with full military honors at the Riverside National Cemetery, Riverside, California, on September 24, 2004.

In recognition of his service, Daclan was posthumously awarded United States citizenship, as well as the Bronze Star and Purple Heart.

Edgar is survived by his parents, Edgar Sr. and Gertrude; and sisters Cristine, Ira, Sheila, Aileen, and Iris.

NORMAN DARLING

Died: April 29, 2004
Branch: U.S. Army

Private First Class Norman Darling died on April 29, 2004, in Baghdad, Iraq. He was one of eight Soldiers killed by a suicide car bomb as his unit conducted a dismounted patrol sweep for IEDs. The 29-year-old medic was assigned to the 4th Battalion, 27th Field Artillery Regiment, 1st Armored Division in Baumholder, Germany. Family and friends said their final farewells on May 10, 2004, when he was buried at Massachusetts National Cemetery.

Darling was awarded the Bronze Star and Purple Heart, in addition to a certificate of U.S. citizenship. He leaves behind his wife, Kimberly; adoring daughter, Camryn; proud parents, Sidney and Madlyn; and siblings, Jaye, Christopher, Rodney, Cindy, and Crystal.

MICHAEL A. DIRAIMONDO

Died: January 8, 2004
Branch: U.S. Army

Sergeant Michael A. DiRaimondo was killed, 8 January, 2004, when the UH-60 MEDVAC Helicopter on which he was serving as Flight Medic was shot down near Fallujah, Iraq. He was assigned to the 571st Medical Company, home stationed at Fort Carson, Colorado, in support of Operation Iraqi Freedom. Also killed were three other crewmembers from the 571st and five Soldiers being transported to a medical facility in Baghdad. A memorial service was held by the 571st Medical Company on January 11, 2004. His body was then flown home to Simi Valley, California, where he was buried in Assumption Cemetery.

To honor his memory, his parents established the Michael A. DiRaimondo Foundation to provide academic aid to young men and women who want to train as paramedics. Michael is survived by his parents, Tony and Carol; and his sisters, Dawn and Danielle.

PETER G. ENOS

Died: April 9, 2004
Branch: U.S. Army

Sergeant Peter G. Enos lost his life on April 9, 2004, in Bayji, Iraq, while supporting Operation Iraqi Freedom. The 24-year-old Army Medic was killed when the patrol vehicle he was riding in was hit by a rocket propelled grenade. He was assigned to the 1st Battalion, 7th Field Artillery Regiment, 1st Infantry Division in Schweinfurt, Germany. Family and close friends celebrated his life in a private ceremony before honoring his wishes and laying him in his final resting spot with full military honors in Arlington National Cemetery.

Enos was posthumously promoted from Specialist to Sergeant. He was also awarded the Bronze Star for Valor, the Purple Heart, and the Combat Medical Badge. Peter is survived by his wife, Shannon; his son, Marcus; and his parents, Joe and Deborah.

BILLY GOMEZ

Died: October 27, 2004
Branch: U.S. Army

Corporal Billy Gomez died on October 27, 2004, at Landstuhl Regional Medical Center, Germany. He was fatally wounded on October 20 when the vehicle he was riding in hit an improvised land mine. The 25-year-old Combat Medic was assigned to the 25th Infantry Division, Schofield Barracks, Hawaii. He was serving with Headquarters and Headquarters Company of the 2nd Battalion, 27th Infantry Regiment and was in Afghanistan supporting Operation Enduring Freedom. Members of his unit gathered to pay their final respects to their fallen comrade on October 30, 2004, at Forward Operation Base Orgun-E in Afghanistan.

When the family learned of Billy's fatal accident, they immediately gathered in Germany to join their son during his last moments. His mother recalls, "I was there for the beginning of his life, and I was there in the end. My heart aches for all the things he will not experience, but I truly believe that he is still here with us in our hearts and spirit."

Billy is survived by his mother, Maria; his brothers, Joey and Mark; his sister Debbie; and his nephew, Anthony.

MELISSA J. HOBART

Died: June 6, 2004
Branch: U.S. Army

Private First Class Melissa J. Hobart lost her life on June 6, 2004, while in Iraq supporting Operation Iraqi Freedom. She was on guard duty in Baghdad, Iraq, when she collapsed. The 22-year-old Combat Medic was assigned to E Company, 215th Forward Support Battalion, 1st Cavalry Division out of Fort Hood, Texas. More than 100 family and friends gathered at the Summerville Presbyterian Church in Summerville, South Carolina, on June 10, 2004, to honor her. She was laid to rest in Connecticut, where most of her family resides.

Melissa is survived by her daughter, Alexis; her father, Gary; and her brothers, Stephen and Gary.

AARON N. HOLLEYMAN
Died: August 30, 2004
Branch: U.S. Army

Staff Sergeant Aaron N. Holleyman lost his life while conducting combat patrols in Khutayiah, Iraq, on August 30, 2004, when the vehicle he was riding in hit an IED. Supporting Operation Iraqi Freedom, the 26-year-old Special Forces Medical Sergeant was assigned to the 1st Battalion, 5th Special Forces Group out of Fort Campbell, Kentucky. He had been in Iraq on his second tour for less than two months at the time of his death. On September 7, 2004, his funeral took place at the Trinity Baptist Church in Carthage, Mississippi, after which he was buried with full military honors in Monticello Baptist Church Cemetery.

Aaron is survived by his parents, Ross and Glenda; three children, Erin, Shelby, and Zach; sister, Kelly and brother, Daniel.

PHILIP A. JOHNSON, JR.
Died: January 8, 2004
Branch: U.S. Army

Chief Warrant Officer Two Philip A. Johnson, Jr., was killed on January 8, 2004, when an enemy missile near Fallujah, Iraq, shot down the helicopter he was piloting. He was assigned to the 571st Medical Company, home stationed with the 3rd Armored Cavalry Regiment at Fort Carson, Colorado. Also killed were three other crew members from the 571st and five Soldiers being transported to a medical facility in Baghdad. Johnson is buried in Arlington National Cemetery in Arlington, Virginia.

Philip is survived by his wife, Melissa; his parents, Philip and Barbara; and his brothers, Matthew and Peter.

GUSSIE M. JONES

Died: March 7, 2004
Branch: U.S. Army

Captain Gussie M. Jones, an Army Nurse Corps officer assigned to the 31st Combat Support Hospital in Baghdad, Iraq, died of cardiac arrest on March 7, 2004, in support of Operation Iraqi Freedom. Even though Jones was exhausted from working a full shift, she immediately answered the call when an urgent request came in for assistance from another unit. After funeral services on March 15, 2004, at Saint Mark Baptist Church, Little Rock, Arkansas, Jones was buried in Arkansas State Veterans Cemetery.

Gussie leaves behind her loving extended family and the brothers and sisters she served with.

MICHAEL G. KARR, JR.

Died: March 31, 2004
Branch: U.S. Army

Specialist Michael G. Karr, Jr., an Army Medic assigned to the 1st Engineer Battalion, 1st Brigade Combat Team, 1st Infantry Division, Fort Riley, Kansas, was killed in action on March 31, 2004, with four other Soldiers in Iraq. His armored personnel carrier ran over a bomb, possibly detonated by remote control. A Mass of Christian Burial was held on April 8, 2004, at the First United Methodist Church, Mt. Vernon, Texas, followed by a military service at the Dallas-Fort Worth National Cemetery. In June 2004, a ceremony was held at Arlington National Cemetery, honoring Karr and the four other Soldiers who died alongside him. Their common grave is marked by a single gravestone that includes all five names.

Michael is survived by his mother, Kim; his father Greg; his sisters, Michele and Erin; and a large extended family.

IAN D. MANUEL
Died: January 8, 2004
Branch: U.S. Army

Chief Warrant Officer Two Ian D. Manuel was killed on January 8, 2004, when an enemy missile shot down the helicopter he was piloting near Fallujah, Iraq. He was assigned to the 571st Medical Company, 3rd Armored Cavalry Regiment at Fort Carson, Colorado.

Manuel's father served in the Navy and his grandfather flew combat missions in World War II. This legacy of service motivated Manuel to fly in the military. He entered the Army Warrant Officer Program and then completed flight training to become an Army Aviator. After receiving his aviator wings, he reported to the 571st Medical Company at Fort Carson.

Ian is survived by his father, Brice; and his mother Tita. He is also survived by his fiancée Jill.

FERNANDO A. MENDEZ-ACEVES
Died: April 6, 2004
Branch: U.S. Navy

Petty Officer Third Class Fernando A. Mendez-Aceves was shot and killed April 6, 2004, while tending to another Marine who had been shot during combat in Fallujah, Iraq. The 27-year-old Hospital Corpsman was assigned to the Naval Medical Center San Diego, 1st Marine Division, in San Diego, California. His body was cremated, and his ashes, together with those of his great-grandfather, rest in Chula Vista, California.

Fernando is survived by his mother, Sandra; and his three brothers, Rodrigo, Enrique, and Kenneth.

HARRISON J. MEYER

Died: November 26, 2004
Branch: U.S. Army

Private First Class Harrison J. Meyer, an Army Medic, was killed in action on November 26, 2004, in Ar Ramadi, Iraq. He and four other Soldiers were wounded by a machine gunner while crossing a street. Meyer was able to find cover despite being shot in the calf and abdomen, yet, with utter disregard for his own safety, he ran into the street to move his wounded comrades to cover. Shot again several times, he died. Meyer served with the 3rd Platoon, D Company, 1st Battalion, 503rd Infantry Regiment, 2nd Brigade Combat Team, 2nd Infantry Division of Camp Howze, Korea, in support of Operation Iraqi Freedom. He was buried with full military honors at Resurrection Cemetery in Columbus, Ohio.

Meyer was posthumously awarded the Silver Star, the Bronze Star and the Purple Heart. He is survived by his parents, William and Debra.

CHARLES E. ODUMS, II

Died: May 30, 2004
Branch: U.S. Army

Specialist Charles E. Odums, II, an Army Medic, died in action on May 30, 2004, when his convoy hit an explosive device in Baghdad, Iraq. Odums was attached to the Headquarters Company, 1st Battalion, 8th Cavalry Regiment, 1st Cavalry Division out of Fort Hood, Texas. On June 9, 2004, funeral services were conducted at the Ebenezer Baptist Church in Sandusky, Ohio, after which hundreds of family members, friends, military veterans, townspeople, and service members watched as his casket was carried by military detail to an open marble pavilion in Oakland Cemetery. Many held flags and some saluted or stood with hand over heart as the Soldier's funeral procession passed.

Charles is survived by his wife, Melanie; his parents, Charles and Annie; a brother, Robert; and sisters, Janel, Sophia, Candenisa, and Tashica.

TONY B. OLAES

Died: September 20, 2004
Branch: U.S. Army

Staff Sergeant Tony B. Olaes was killed on September 20, 2004. The 30-year-old Special Forces Combat Medic was in Shkin, Afghanistan, supporting his country in Operation Enduring Freedom when enemy forces using small-arms fire and rockets ambushed his patrol vehicle. Staff Sergeant Olaes was assigned to the 2nd Battalion, 3rd Special Forces Group out of Fort Bragg, North Carolina. Family and friends gathered on September 29, 2004, to honor their beloved hero at the Sandifer Funeral Home Chapel in Westminster, South Carolina, followed by burial services with full military honors at Heritage Memorial Gardens.

Olaes is survived by his wife, Tammy; and his three children, Maverick, McKenzie, and Alec.

JUSTIN B. ONWORDI

Died: August 2, 2004
Branch: U.S. Army

Specialist Justin B. Onwordi, an Army Medic attached to Headquarters and Headquarters Company, 2nd Battalion, 12th Armored Cavalry Regiment, 1st Cavalry Division out of Fort Hood, Texas, gave his life for his adopted country on August 2, 2004, when an improvised explosive device (IED) detonated near the vehicle in which he was patrolling in Baghdad, Iraq. He had served as a Combat Medic in Iraq since January 2004, providing lifesaving care to wounded Soldiers and patrolling the dangerous byways of Baghdad. Justin was buried on August 19, 2004, with full military honors, at Montlawn Memorial Park, Raleigh, North Carolina. The funeral had been delayed so that family members from Nigeria could travel to attend the ceremony.

Justin, one of four children, was a native of Lagos, Nigeria. Since childhood, he knew his life's path was in the military. Justin was a cadet in the Nigerian military throughout his high school years. He emigrated from Nigeria to the United States in July 2000, intent on joining the military. Six months later, he enlisted in the Army and trained as a Combat Medic at Fort Sam Houston, San Antonio, Texas.

Justin is survived by his wife, Monique; his son Jonathan; his mother, Virginia; and his two sisters, Jacqueline and Martina.

TYLER D. PREWITT
Died: September 28, 2004
Branch: U.S. Army

Sergeant Tyler D. Prewitt an Army Medic assigned to the 2nd Battalion, 2nd Infantry Regiment, 1st Infantry Division out of Vilseck, Germany, died at Landstuhl Regional Medical Center in Germany on September 28, 2004, from injuries sustained in Baqubah, Iraq, in support of Operation Iraqi Freedom. An armor-piercing rocket cut through the side of his vehicle. As the only medic at the scene, Prewitt calmly instructed other fighters how to treat all the wounds, including his injury, before he lost consciousness. Even after death, Prewitt was still saving lives: his organs were donated to seven terminally-ill people in Germany. Funeral services were held for Prewitt on October 7, 2004, at Palmcroft Baptist Church in Phoenix, Arizona. He was buried with military honors at the National Memorial Cemetery of Arizona.

Tyler is survived by his parents, Tim and Jonnie; and two older brothers, Richie and Chad.

OMEAD H. RAZANI
Died: August 27, 2004
Branch: U.S. Army

Specialist Omead H. Razani, an Army Medic assigned to Headquarters and Headquarters Company, 1st Battalion, 506th Infantry Regiment, 2nd Brigade Combat Team, 2nd Infantry Division out of Camp Greaves, South Korea, died on August 27, 2004. Razani was shot as he rendered aid to a Soldier injured in a firefight with Iraqi insurgents. He was the first Iranian-American Soldier to fall in Iraq.

Razani enlisted in the Army immediately after high school and trained as a Combat Medic. A native of California, Omead was only 19 years old when he died. His inspiration to seek training in the medical field was his father, a psychiatrist who had emigrated from Iran.

Omead is survived by his mother, Shala; his father, Javed; and his sister, Nooshin.

MATTHEW J. SANDRI
Died: March 20, 2004
Branch: U.S. Army

Sergeant Matthew J. Sandri, an Army Medic attached to Charlie Company, 82nd Forward Support Battalion, Fort Bragg, North Carolina, was killed in action on March 20, 2004, while supporting Operation Iraqi Freedom. He died as a result of injuries sustained in a rocket attack on the medical facility where he worked at Forward Operating Base Sainte, near Fallujah, Iraq. The attack also killed Lieutenant Colonel Mark Taylor, a physician with the 82nd Airborne Division, and wounded five Soldiers and one Sailor. Sandri's memorial service was held in the town's high school gym, the only place large enough to hold the number of mourners who attended, and he was buried in Saint Edwards Cemetery, Shamokin, Pennsylvania.

Matt is survived by his parents Bob and Annette.

JEFFREY R. SHAVER
Died: May 12, 2004
Branch: U.S. Army

Sergeant Jeffrey R. Shaver, an Army National Guard Medic assigned to the 1st Battalion, 161st Infantry Regiment, 81st Brigade Combat Team, Army National Guard out of Spokane, Washington, was killed when an explosive device struck his vehicle on May 12, 2004, in Baghdad, Iraq. He had been involved in a humanitarian mission at a civilian clinic at the time. On May 29, 2004, a military funeral was held at the Tahoma National Cemetery, Maple Valley,

Washington, following his memorial service. An eternal testament to Shaver's motto of life, engraved on his headstone, is "LOVE AND LIVE LIFE WITH PASSION!"

Jeff is survived by his parents, John and Jane; his sisters, Gwen and Sakura; and his fiancée, Charity.

CHARLES R. SOLTES, JR.
Died: October 13, 2004
Branch: U.S. Army

Major Charles R. Soltes, Jr., was killed on October 13, 2004, in Mosul, Iraq. Soltes was returning from a meeting with Iraqi health officials at a local hospital when a suicide car bomber drove into his vehicle, killing him and another American and wounding five others. Soltes was assigned as a preventive medicine officer to the 426th Civil Affairs Battalion out of Upland, California. He was buried at the Pacific View Memorial Park, Corona del Mar, California.

Charles is survived by his wife, Sally; his sons, Ryan and Brandon; his parents, Charles and Nancy; his brother, Jeff; and his sister, Carolyn.

ADRIAN B. SZWEC
Died: April 12, 2004
Branch: U.S. Navy

United States Navy Commander Adrian B. Szwec died on April 12, 2004, as a result of a non-combat related incident. A Navy physician, he was assigned to the Naval Hospital, Guantanamo Bay, Cuba, in support of Operation Enduring Freedom. Fellow comrades gathered at the Guantanamo Bay base chapel on April 16, 2004, to remember and honor their fallen Sailor.

MARK D. TAYLOR
Died: March 20, 2004
Branch: U.S. Army

Lieutenant Colonel Mark D. Taylor died from wounds received during a rocket attack on March 20, 2004, in Fallujah, Iraq, in support of Operation Iraqi Freedom. As a physician assigned to forward surgical team of the 782nd Main Support Battalion, 82nd Airborne Division, he was retrieving wounded Soldiers near his base when the attack occurred. Mark was buried at Cherokee Memorial Cemetery in Lodi, California.

Mark is survived by his parents, Doug and Roberta; and his son, Connor.

LEE D. TODACHEENE
Died: April 6, 2004
Branch: U.S. Army

Sergeant Lee D. Todacheene, an Army Medic attached to the 1st Battalion, 77th Armor Regiment, 1st Infantry Division out of Schweinfurt, Germany, was killed on April 6, 2004, while on guard duty in Balad, Iraq. After a funeral mass was celebrated ay Saint Isabelle Church in Lukachukai, Arizona, Todacheene was buried in Saint Isabelle Community Cemetery on April 12, 2004. He was the first Navajo tribe member to be killed in the Iraq war.

Lee is survived by his wife, Jacqueline; his sons, Cody and Dylan; his parents Melvin and Alberta; his brother, Rydell; and his sister, Donna,

ROY A. WOOD
Died: January 9, 2004
Branch: U.S. Army

Sergeant Roy A. Wood died on January 9, 2004, when the vehicle he was traveling in near Kabul, Afghanistan, hit another vehicle as it was returning in a convoy from Qalat to Bagram Air Base. He was evacuated to a combat support hospital at Bagram Air Base, where he succumbed to his wounds. Wood was assigned to C Company, 3rd Battalion, 20th Special Forces Group, Army National Guard based in Starke, Florida, in support of Operation Enduring Freedom. He was buried in the Georgia Veterans Memorial Cemetery in Milledgeville, Georgia, on January 20, 2004.

Roy is survived by his wife, Hana; his son, Roy, and his daughter, Caroline; his parents, Julia and Calvin; and his two brothers and two sisters.

JULIAN WOODS

Died: November 10, 2004
Branch: U.S. Navy

Petty Officer Third Class Julian Woods sacrificed his life for his country while fighting beside the Marines he was committed to saving in support of Operation Iraqi Freedom. He died as a result of hostile fire on November 10, 2004, in Fallujah, Iraq. The 22-year-old was assigned to the 3rd Marine Division Detachment, Marine Corps Base Hawaii. Several hundred friends and relatives gathered to honor their fallen hero November 22, 2004, at the Second Missionary Baptist Church in Jacksonville, Florida. He was laid to rest with full military honors in Riverside Memorial Park.

Serving in his fourth year of a six-year enlistment, Woods followed in his father's and older brother's footsteps when he joined the Navy shortly after high school.

Julian is survived by his mother and father, Carolyn and Julius; his daughter, Israel; and his brothers, Octavius, Julius, David and Alexis.

CESAR O. BAEZ

Died: June 15, 2005
Branch: U.S. Navy

U.S. Navy Petty Officer Second Class Cesar O. Baez perished from wounds incurred from enemy small-arms fire on June 15, 2005, near Ramadi, Iraq. The 37-year-old was a Hospital Corpsman assigned to the 2nd Marine Division, II Marine Expeditionary Force based at Camp Lejeune, North Carolina. His younger brother Marine Staff Sergeant Roger Baez, who was stationed in Germany, escorted Cesar's remains from Dover Air Force Base, Delaware, home to California.

Baez committed many years of his life to service on behalf of his country. Originally, he joined the United States Marine Corps and served in that capacity for four years. After finishing his stint with the Marines, Baez enlisted in the U.S. Navy and actively served in that branch for ten years, up to the time of his death.

Cesar is survived by his wife, Rosanna; his children Isabel, Sydney, Suzy, and newborn son; his parents Cesar and Bernardina; and his brother Marine Staff Sergeant Roger Baez.

TAYLOR J. BURK
Died: January 26, 2005
Branch: U.S. Army

Specialist Taylor Burk died January 26, 2005, when an improvised explosive device detonated near his HMMWV in Baghdad, Iraq. Specialist Burk was serving his second tour in Iraq and was assigned to the U.S. Army's 1st Battalion, 8th Cavalry Regiment, 1st Cavalry Division out of Fort Hood, Texas. The 21-year-old Medic, hit in the neck by shrapnel, died clutching his commander's hand and surrounded by his friends. He is buried at Memorial Parke Cemetery in Amarillo, Texas.

Nine months earlier, in April of 2004, Specialist Burk was hit in the foot by gunfire during a nighttime patrol. Another Soldier, Private Joseph Bridges, was hit in the face and thigh, almost severing his leg. During that incident, Burk worked to save Bridges' life, even as enemy gunfire continued, striking the vehicle and Bridges once again. Burk continued to hover over him, screaming in Bridges' ear that he was not going to die. Bridges was then rushed to a nearby medical facility. Burk's quick action, and insistence on driving the wounded Soldier to a surgical hospital in an unfamiliar part of Baghdad, earned him the Bronze Star, Purple Heart, and Combat Medical Badge.

Taylor is survived by his parents, Tracy and Tim; sister Julie; and brother Wheeler.

DAMION G. O. CAMPBELL
Died: August 26, 2005
Branch: U.S. Army

Staff Sergeant Damion Campbell was killed on August 26, 2005, when an improvised explosive device detonated near his vehicle during a combat patrol in Khayr Kot, Afghanistan. The 23-year-old Combat Medic was assigned to the 1st Battalion, 508th Parachute Infantry Regiment, 173rd Airborne Brigade Combat Team based in Vincenza, Italy, supporting Operation Enduring Freedom. Campbell was buried in Garrison Forest Veterans Cemetery in Owings Mills, Maryland.

Damion leaves behind his mother, Donna; father, Yandell; brothers, Paul and Nicholas; and sisters, Yandeen and Racheal.

RICHARD M. CRANE
Died: February 8, 2005
Branch: U.S. Army

Specialist Richard M. Crane died in his sleep on February 8, 2005, while serving in Kandahar, Afghanistan, in support of Operation Enduring Freedom. Specialist Crane served as a Surgical Technician and Combat Medic in the Army Reserve and was assigned to the 325th Field Hospital, Independence, Missouri. The 25-year-old husband and father of three was just a month shy of returning to the United States. Family and friends said their farewells on February 18, 2005, at Broadview Christian Church in Kansas City, after which he was laid to rest in Mound Grove Cemetery in Independence, Missouri.

In addition to his beloved wife, Liana, Richard leaves three adoring sons, Mateo, Michael, and Ricky; his parents, Mike and Susan; and sister, Madison.

ALLAN M. CUNDANGAN ESPIRITU

Died: November 1, 2005
Branch: U.S. Navy

Petty Officer Second Class Allan M. Cundangan Espiritu was killed on November 1, 2005, by an improvised explosive device in the vicinity of Ar Ramadi, Iraq. Espiritu was a Hospital Corpsman assigned to the 7th Engineer Support Battalion, 2nd Force Support Group of the Marine Expeditionary Force based at Camp Pendleton, California. He was on his second tour of duty in Iraq and had volunteered for service with an Explosive Disposal Unit, passing up safer duties so he could be where he was needed. He was buried at the Ivy Lawn Memorial Park in Ventura, California.

Allan was born in the Philippines but immigrated to California with his parents in 1981. He played football at Channel Island High School in Oxnard, California, and graduated in 1995.

Allan is survived by his wife, Erika (also a Navy Corpsman); his daughters, Alissa, Melanie and Alexy; and his parents and two brothers.

RAY M. FUHRMANN, II

Died: August 18, 2005
Branch: U.S. Army

Specialist Ray M. Fuhrmann, II, died August 18, 2005, when an improvised explosive device detonated near his vehicle in Samarra, Iraq, while he was serving in support of Operation Iraqi Freedom. Fuhrmann was helping to escort Explosive Ordnance Disposal Soldiers from the site of another improvised explosive device. Three other Soldiers died with him. Specialist Fuhrmann, 28 years old, was assigned to the 3rd Battalion, 69th Armored Regiment, 1st Brigade Combat Team, 3rd Infantry Division out of Fort Stewart, Georgia. Fuhrmann served with the Army Rangers during the initial invasion of Iraq. He told relatives that he had been involved in ten of the eleven major battles during that invasion. At the time of his death, he was on his second tour in Iraq. The Medic who cared for him the day he was killed especially remembers his bravery. He recalls that Fuhrmann was more concerned for the other Medics than for himself.

Ray is survived by his wife, Tylea; his father Michael; and his brother Tyler.

SEAN P. GRIMES
Died: March 4, 2005
Branch: U.S. Army

Captain Sean P. Grimes was killed on March 4, 2005, in Ramadi, Iraq, when an improvised explosive device exploded near his vehicle, killing him and three other Soldiers. He was a Physician Assistant assigned as the Assistant Battalion Surgeon to the 1st Battalion, 9th Infantry Regiment, 2nd Brigade Combat Team, 2nd Infantry Division supporting Operation Iraqi Freedom. Grimes was the first Army Physician Assistant to be killed in action in Iraq. He was buried in Saint Charles Cemetery, Farmingdale, New York.

For his service, Grimes was awarded the Bronze Star, Purple Heart, and the Morris County (New Jersey) Distinguished Service Medal. Sean is survived by his parents, Donald and Mary; two siblings, Mary and Donald, Jr.; and numerous friends and family.

GARY R. HARPER, JR.
Died: October 9, 2005
Branch: U.S. Army

Staff Sergeant Gary R. Harper, Jr., died on October 9, 2005, in Baghdad, Iraq, from wounds he sustained when Islamic insurgents attacked his recon mission while he was supporting his country in Operation Iraqi Freedom. The 29-year-old was serving as a Special Forces Medic with the 2nd Battalion, 5th Special Forces Group out of Fort Campbell, Kentucky. A memorial service in Harper's honor was held at Fort Campbell, Kentucky, on October 14, 2005. He was buried with full military honors in Arlington National Cemetery, Arlington, Virginia. Several months later, on December 10, 2005, 200 mourners attended a second ceremony held in his hometown of Virden, Illinois.

Gary's survivors include his wife, Danielle; his daughter, Madison; two sons, Tristen and Gabrian; his mother Linda; and two brothers and a sister.

MATTHEW J. HOLLEY
Died: November 15, 2005
Branch: U.S. Army

Specialist Matthew J. Holley was one of four Soldiers who died on November 15, 2005, in a bomb blast during combat operations in Taji, Iraq. The 21-year-old was supporting Operation Iraqi Freedom and was assigned to the 1st Battalion, 320th Field Artillery Regiment, 101st Airborne Division out of Fort Campbell, Kentucky. Holley was buried at Glen Abbey Memorial Park in Bonita, California.

Matthew is survived by his parents, John and Stacey.

JOHN D. HOUSE
Died: January 26, 2005
Branch: U.S. Navy

Petty Officer Third Class John D. House, a devoted Navy Corpsman assigned to the Naval Medical Clinic Hawaii, Marine Corps Units Detachment in Pearl Harbor, lost his life on January 26, 2005, when a Marine Corps transport helicopter crashed during a sand storm near Rutbah, Iraq, killing him and 30 other Marines. The 28-year-old was attached to C Company, 1st Battalion, 3rd Marine Regiment and was serving on his second mission to Iraq. Although originally scheduled to return to the United States in July 2004, he chose to remain in Iraq because of a shortage of Corpsman and was set to return to Hawaii 19 days after his death. House was laid to rest in Simi Valley, California.

A memorial service was held February 3, 2005, at Pearl Harbor Memorial Chapel, with over 500 people in attendance, including ranking Navy and Marine Corps officials.

John is survived by his wife, Melanie; his son, James; and his parents, Susan and Larry.

TRICIA L. JAMESON
Died: July 14, 2005
Branch: U.S. Army

Sergeant First Class Tricia Jameson died July 14, 2005, when a roadside explosive detonated near her ambulance in Trebil, Iraq. As her ambulance approached to aid wounded Marines who had been attacked by a roadside bomb, another explosive detonated, killing Jameson. Jameson was stationed at a 313th Medical Company remote site for the Lincoln, Nebraska, National Guard. Jameson was buried with full military honors at Bohemian National Cemetery in Omaha, Nebraska.

Tricia is survived by her mother, Patricia; her brother, Robert; and her fiancé, Mike.

ALLEN C. JOHNSON
Died: April 26, 2005
Branch: U.S. Army

Sergeant First Class Allen C. Johnson died April 26, 2005, in Khanaqin, Afghanistan, while conducting a combat patrol. His unit came under small-arms fire and Johnson managed to flank Taliban forces in order to free his Operational Detachment A Team, which was pinned down by enemy fire. He drew concentrated fire from the enemy and his team was able to maneuver from the ambush. Johnson was hit and subsequently died of his wounds. The 31-year-old Special Forces Medical Sergeant was assigned to the 1st Battalion, 7th Special Forces Group in Fort Bragg, North Carolina, in support of Operation Enduring Freedom. His funeral was held on May 4, 2005, at the New Life Church in Corning, California, after which he was laid to rest in Los Molinos Cemetery in Los Milinos, California.

Allen is survived by his mother, Adriaantje; his father, Gary; his wife Vanessa; and three children, Stacy, Joshua, and Naomi.

JUDE R. JONAUS

Died: September 6, 2005
Branch: U.S. Army

Staff Sergeant Jude R. Jonaus was killed September 6, 2005, when a roadside explosion caused his vehicle to roll over. At the time of the incident, Jonaus and another Soldier were performing duties as the brigade headquarters personal security team in support of Operation Iraqi Freedom. Jonaus was a Pharmacy Technician assigned to the Brigade Troops Battalion, Division Support Brigade, 3rd Infantry Division out of Fort Stewart, Georgia. He was laid to rest in Florida National Cemetery in Bushnell, Florida.

Jude is survived by his loving devoted parents, Gernessoit and Amenia; his six siblings; and extended family and friends.

CHRISTOPHER M. KATZENBERGER

Died: August 9, 2005
Branch: U.S. Army

Specialist Christopher Katzenberger died August 9, 2005, of injuries received when an improvised explosive device detonated near his vehicle near Bagram Air Base in Afghanistan. He was assigned to C Company, 2nd Battalion, 504th Parachute Infantry Regiment, 82nd Airborne Division out of Fort Bragg, North Carolina, in support of Operation Enduring Freedom. He was buried with full military honors in Jefferson Barracks National Cemetery in St. Louis, Missouri.

Chris is survived by his parents, Michael and Kathleen; his sister, Amanda; and his grandparents, Al and Minnie.

AARON A. KENT

Died: April 23, 2005
Branch: U.S. Navy

Navy Hospital Corpsman Aaron A. Kent was killed on April 23, 2005, when a roadside bomb exploded near his vehicle during combat operations near Fallujah, Iraq. Kent was assigned to the 2nd Marine Division, II Marine Expeditionary Force out of Camp Lejeune, North Carolina, in support of Operation Iraqi Freedom. Funeral services were held May 4, 2005, at New Hope Community Church in Portland, Oregon, and Kent was laid to rest at the Williamette National Cemetery.

Aaron is survived by his parents, Gary and Lara, along with a sister, Mikaela, and brother, Mitchell.

JAMES C. KESINGER
Died: December 13, 2005
Branch: U.S. Army

Specialist James C. Kesinger was killed on December 13, 2005, when an improvised explosive device detonated near his vehicle in Taji, Iraq, while he was conducting combat operations. Kesinger was 32 years old and on his second tour in Iraq in support of Operation Iraqi Freedom. He was assigned to the 2nd Battalion, 70th Armor Regiment 3rd Brigade Combat Team, 1st Armored Division out of Fort Riley, Kansas. During his memorial service Kessinger's father Cliff, who served in the Vietnam War, saluted not only his son but all service members: "You are all my heroes." He was laid to rest in Memory Gardens in Corpus Christi, Texas.

Kesinger served one year in the National Guard before enlisting in the Reserve in 2002. His first deployment to Iraq was in January 2003. In 2004, he became active duty. He had volunteered to leave his company for a second tour in Iraq to join another company in desperate need of Medics.

Friends and family remember a man small in stature, but great of heart. James was a caring and devoted family man with a bright smile and a winning sense of humor. He always tried to ease the fears of others and bring joy to those around him. In high school in Zapata, Texas, James ran track, played football, and was in the school band. He was also one of two male cheerleaders. In addition, he participated in 4-H and trained to become a black belt in Taekwondo. Friends from school remember his sense of humor and witty remarks.

James met his wife, Sanjuana Zuniga, online. They developed a relationship while he was stationed in Iraq on his first tour in 2003. The comforting words on the screen sent thousands of miles went straight to their hearts. On his two-week leave James and Sanjuana met in person for the first time. By the end of his leave they were married. While on his second tour in Iraq, in the summer of 2005, he came home on leave for 15 days and they welcomed their first child. Although James was able to meet his son before he returned to Iraq, Jared will never know his father except through pictures.

James is survived by his wife, Sanjuana, and their son, Jared; five children, Justice, Christian, Brianna, Meredith, and Megan; parents Cliff and Deanna; and his sisters, Tanya and Tina.

BRYAN W. LARGE
Died: October 3, 2005
Branch: U.S. Army

Sergeant Bryan W. Large was killed during combat operations in Haglaniyah, Iraq, on October 3, 2005. The 31-year-old Soldier was lead Medic of D Company, 3rd Battalion, 504th Parachute Infantry Regiment, 82nd Airborne Division out of Fort Bragg, North Carolina. He was in the vanguard of a major offensive called Operation River Gate when an improvised explosive device detonated near his vehicle. Two other Soldiers were also killed in the blast. He was buried with full military honors at Chestnut Hill Memorial Park in Cuyahoga Falls, Ohio.

Large joined the Army Reserve after the 9/11 attacks and became a Paratrooper and a Medic. He was on his second tour in Iraq, having served his first tour in 2004. He also served in Afghanistan in 2003. Large planned to become a firefighter and paramedic after serving in the Army.

Bryan is survived by his daughters Kylie and Devan; his parents, Linda and Larry; and his sister Michelle.

LEE A. LEWIS, JR.
Died: March 18, 2005
Branch: U.S. Army

Private First Class Lee A. Lewis, Jr., was killed March 18, 2005, when his patrol came under attack in Sadr City, Iraq. The 28-year-old Medic served with the 3rd Battalion, 15th Infantry Regiment, 3rd Infantry Division out of Fort Stewart, Georgia, in support of Operation Iraqi Freedom. He was the 125th fatality of Operation Iraqi Freedom to be buried at Arlington National Cemetery, Arlington, Virginia.

Lee is survived by his wife, Telia, and his daughter, Justina; as well as his parents, Lee and Elvena.

ROBERT N. MARTENS
Died: September 6, 2005
Branch: U.S. Navy

Hospital Corpsman Robert N. Martens of Queen Creek, Arizona, lost his life due to injuries he received when the vehicle he was riding in during a night patrol rolled over in Al Qaim, Iraq, on September 6, 2005, just 10 days after arriving in Iraq. Martens was assigned to the 2nd Marine Division at Camp Lejeune, North Carolina. The 20-year-old Corpsman is buried at City of Mesa Cemetery in Mesa, Arizona.

For his heroic service, Martens was awarded the Feet Marine Force Pin. In addition to his parents, Rob and Maria; his wife Erin, and daughter Riley Jo, Robert leaves behind his sister, Bobbie; his brother, Matthew; and many other friends and family.

STEPHEN M. MCGOWAN
Died: March 4, 2005
Branch: U.S. Army

Corporal Stephen M. McGowan was killed on March 4, 2005, when an improvised explosive device detonated near his patrol in Ramadi, Iraq. The 26-year-old was assigned to the 1st Battalion, 9th

Infantry Regiment, 2nd Brigade Combat Team, 2nd Infantry Division out of Camp Hovey, Korea, to support Operation Iraqi Freedom. He had volunteered to go to Iraq so that a fellow Medic with children would not have to go. McGowan was buried with full military honors in Arlington National Cemetery.

McGowan's honors and decorations include the Combat Medic Badge. He is survived by his mother, Bobbie; and his sister, Michaela.

JAMES H. MILLER, IV
Died: January 30, 2005
Branch: U.S. Army

Private First Class James H. Miller, IV, died on January 30, 2005, when an improvised explosive device detonated near his vehicle while he was guarding a polling station in Ramadi during Iraqi elections. The 22-year-old Medic was assigned to the Army's 1st Battalion, 503rd Infantry Regiment, 2nd Infantry Division out of Camp Casey, South Korea. Miller completed his basic training at Fort Sill, Oklahoma, before training as a Medic at Fort Sam Houston, Texas. He deployed to South Korea and served there for several months before receiving his assignment to support Operation Iraqi Freedom.

James leaves behind his proud father, James, and his two brothers.

LAWRENCE E. MORRISON
Died: September 19, 2005
Branch: U.S. Army

Sergeant First Class Lawrence E. Morrison died on September 19, 2005, in Taji, Iraq, of injuries he sustained when an improvised explosive device detonated near his vehicle. The 45-year-old Medic was a reservist supporting Operation Iraqi Freedom, assigned to the Army Civil Affairs and Psychological Operations Command out of Fort Bragg, North Carolina, and serving with a Marine Corps unit at the time of his death. Friends and family paid their respects on September 30, 2005, at the Keith & Keith Terrace Heights Chapel in

Yakima, Washington, with Morrison's burial in the Terrace Heights Memorial Park.

Lawrence leaves behind a loving and devoted family that includes his wife, Becky; a son, Lawrence; a stepson, Zach; and his father Kenneth.

MARCUS V. MURALLES
Died: June 28, 2005
Branch: U.S. Army

Sergeant First Class Marcus V. Muralles, a Flight Medic assigned to the 160th Special Operations Aviation Regiment (SOAR), was killed in combat in Afghanistan on June 28, 2005, when his helicopter was shot down near Asadabad, Afghanistan. Muralles was part of a task force attempting to rescue a team of four U.S. Navy SEALs trapped deep in enemy controlled territory. Seven other crewmembers and eight SEALs were also killed in the disaster. Muralles was buried in Arlington National Cemetery in Arlington, Virginia, with full military honors.

Muralles enlisted in the U.S. Army in 1994, served as a Combat Medic, and qualified as a Ranger. He left active duty when his tour was complete and went inactive Ready Reserve before going active again in 1998. He requalified as a Medic and was assigned to the elite 75th Ranger Regiment. Subsequently, he qualified as a Special Forces Medic, serving with the regiment until 2003, and performing duty in Iraq and Afghanistan. Muralles was accepted into the 3rd Battalion, 160th SOAR as an Aerial Flight Medic, and in 2005, was again deployed to Afghanistan to support operations against anti-government forces.

Marcus is survived by his wife, Diana; his daughter, Anna; his son, Marcus; his mother Rosemarie; his father, Arturo; and his sister, Cynthia.

RUSSELL H. NAHVI
Died: October 19, 2005
Branch: U.S. Army

Specialist Russell H. Nahvi lost his life on October 9, 2005, when the patrol he had volunteered for was ambushed in Balad, Iraq. The 24-year-old Combat Medic was assigned to the 5th Squadron, 7th Cavalry Regiment, 1st Brigade Combat Team, 3rd Infantry Division out of Fort Stewart, Georgia, in support of Operation Iraqi Freedom. Nahvi's friends and family said their final farewells to him on October 29, 2005, at the Emerald Hills Memorial Chapel, after which he was laid to rest at Emerald Hills Memorial Park in Kennedale, Texas.

Motivated by a hunger for adventure and a longing to fulfill his sense of purpose, in addition to the lure of education benefits, Nahvi joined the Army in 2003. Following in the footsteps of his mother, a nurse, and after seeing the HBO series Band of Brothers, which developed in him a love for the military and the fellowship of Soldiers, Nahvi was inspired to become an Army Combat Medic.

Russell's proud family includes his father, Sam; his mother, Nancy; a sister, Nina; and many extended family and friends.

TIMOTHY R. OSBEY
Died: February 16, 2005
Branch: U.S. Army

Sergeant Timothy R. Osbey lost his life on February 16, 2005, when the vehicle he was riding in rolled into a canal after a section of the road collapsed in Iskandariyah, Iraq. The 29-year-old Combat Medic was assigned to the Army National Guard's 1st Battalion, 155th Infantry Regiment out of McComb, Mississippi. A military honor guard accompanied Osbey back to the United States, where 500 of his family, friends, and community honored their fallen Soldier on February 26, 2005, at the Sherman Missionary Baptist Church in Magnolia, Mississippi, the same church at which he used to sing in the choir. He was laid to rest with military honors in Cook's Cemetery in Pike County, Mississippi.

Sergeant Osbey entered the Mississippi National Guard when he was 18 years old and served 11 years. He deployed to support his country in Operation Iraqi Freedom in January 2005, just a month after being married.

Timothy is survived by his parents, Sherry and Eugene; his wife, Willie Marie; his daughter, Saderia; his sister Michelle, and his brother Tonio.

ROBERT S. PUGH
Died: March 2, 2005
Branch: U.S. Army

Specialist Robert Pugh was killed on March 2, 2005, when his vehicle was hit by an improvised explosive device outside of Iskandariyah, Iraq. Though mortally wounded himself, Pugh instructed a group of Soldiers on how to stop another Soldier's bleeding enough to stabilize him. Pugh's heroic and selfless act saved the wounded Soldier's life. The 25-year-old Combat Medic was assigned to the 1st Battalion, 155th Infantry Regiment, Mississippi Army National Guard out of McComb, Mississippi, in support of Operation Iraqi Freedom. Pugh was laid to rest at Forest Lawn Memory Gardens in Marion, Mississippi.

Robert is remembered by colleagues in and out of the Army as a personable man who had a positive impact on the world around him. Colleague Chris Coffin fondly recalled Robert: "He was a great guy. He would just light up a room and he could lighten the spirit." During Robert's memorial service, he was aptly portrayed as a hero. Reverend Calvin Farmer said, "I remember Robert as being one of the most spiritual kids in my church. He was an example to other youth."

Robert is survived by his wife, Amanda; his mother, Wilma; his father, Glen; his sisters, Jennifer, Tiffany and April; his brothers, Dale and Scotty; and numerous extended family and friends.

MICHAEL T. ROBERTSON
Died: October 25, 2005
Branch: U.S. Army

Sergeant Michael T. Robertson died on October 25, 2005, at Brooke Army Medical Center in San Antonio, Texas. He succumbed to injuries he received when an improvised explosive device detonated near his vehicle on October 17, 2005, in Samarra, Iraq. The 28-year-old Medic was assigned to the 1st Battalion, 15th Infantry Regiment, 3rd Brigade Combat Team, 3rd Infantry Division out of Fort Benning, Georgia. Mourners gathered at the William Temple Church of God, in Houston, Texas, to say their final farewells. He was buried at Houston National Cemetery.

Michael is survived by his wife, Tanya; his son, Xavier; his parents, Barbara and Michael; and his grandparents.

STEVEN F. SIRKO
Died: April 17, 2005
Branch: U.S. Army

Private First Class Steven F. Sirko lost his life on April 17, 2005, in Maqdadiyah, Iraq, in a non-combat related incident. The 20-year-old Combat Medic was supporting his country in Operation Iraqi Freedom and was serving with the 1st Battalion, 30th Infantry Regiment, 3rd Brigade Combat Team, 3rd Infantry Division out of Fort Benning, Georgia. He had been in Iraq for only three months at the time of his death. Friends and family said their final farewells to their beloved Soldier during a funeral Mass held April 23, 2005, at St. Philip the Apostle Catholic Church in Statesville, North Carolina. He was laid to rest with military honors in the Oakwood Cemetery in Statesville.

Steven leaves behind his wife, Virginia; his parents, Steve and Summer; and his sisters, Bridget and Laura.

JEFFREY S. TAYLOR

Died: June 28, 2005
Branch: U.S. Navy

Petty Officer First Class Jeffrey S. Taylor, U.S. Navy, a Hospital Corpsman assigned to SEAL Team Ten, was killed in combat on June 28, 2005, when the helicopter in which he was riding was shot down in Afghanistan. Taylor was part of a task force attempting to rescue a team of four U.S. Navy SEALs trapped deep in enemy controlled territory while supporting Operation Enduring Freedom. Eight U.S. Army crewmembers and seven other SEALs were also killed in the crash. Taylor was buried in Arlington National Cemetery, with full military honors.

He is survived by his wife, Erin; his mother, Gail; his father, John; and his grandmother, Lucille.

CHRISTOPHER W. THOMPSON

Died: October 21, 2005
Branch: U.S. Navy

Petty Officer Third Class Christopher W. Thompson was serving his second tour of duty in Iraq when an improvised explosive device killed him on October 21, 2005. The 25-year-old North Carolina native, who was assigned to Echo Company, 2nd Battalion, 8th Marine Regiment, 2nd Marine Division was conducting combat operations in Al Anbar Province, Iraq. Family and friends honored their beloved son and brother at the Peace Haven Baptist Church in North Wilkesboro, North Carolina; he is buried at Mountlawn Memorial Park.

Chris is survived by his parents, Larry and Geraldine; his two brothers, Jimmy and David; and his grandmother, Statia.

BRIAN A. VAUGHN

Died: June 21, 2005
Branch: U.S. Army

Specialist Brian A. Vaughn died on June 21, 2005, when his unit was attacked by enemy small-arms fire in Ramadi, Iraq. The 23-year-old combat medic was assigned to the 1st Battalion, 9th Infantry Regiment, 2nd Brigade Combat Team, 2nd Infantry Division out of Fort Carson, Colorado. Vaughn's family and friends said their final farewells on June 29, 2005, at First Baptist Church in Trussville, Alabama, after which Vaughn was buried in Jefferson Memorial Gardens in Birmingham, Alabama.

Brian is survived by his mother, Terry; father James; brothers, Adam and Anthony; and sisters Monica, Justine, Felicia, Crystal, and Candy.

JAVIER A. VILLANUEVA

Died: November 24, 2005
Branch: U.S. Army

Specialist Javier A. Villenueva died on November 24, 2005, in Al Asad, Iraq, of wounds he received when a makeshift bomb exploded near his foot patrol in Hit, Iraq, on November 23. Villanueva was assigned to the 2nd Squadron, 11th Armored Cavalry Regiment out of Fort Irwin, California. Friends and family gathered to honor his life on December 3, 2005. He was laid to rest in Waco Memorial Park South in Waco, Texas.

Villanueva joined the Army in September 2003. After completing basic training at Fort Sill, Oklahoma, he reported to Fort Sam Houston in Texas for advanced individual training as a Combat Medic. His first duty station was Fort Irwin, California.

Javier is survived by his wife Felicia; his daughter Taliyah Ann; his parents Cristine and Wilfredo; his brothers David, Carlos, and Wilfredo; and a large circle of family and friends.

KENNETH G. VON RONN

Died: January 6, 2005
Branch: U.S. Army

Sergeant Kenneth G. von Ronn died January 6, 2005, when a roadside bomb exploded under his Bradley fighting vehicle in the village of Awad al-Hussein, north of Baghdad, Iraq. Von Ronn was assigned to Headquarters Company, 1st Battalion, 69th Infantry Regiment, 42nd Infantry Division, Army National Guard out of Newburgh, New York. Six Soldiers from the Louisiana National Guard serving with the 69th Infantry Regiment died in the same incident. Von Ronn was buried on January 15, 2005, with full military honors at Sullivan County Veterans Cemetery in Liberty, New York.

He is survived by his wife, Kira; his parents, Debra and Raymond; his sisters, Gina, Courtney, and Samantha; and a wide circle of friends and family.

THOMAS A. WALLSMITH

Died: October 26, 2005
Branch: U.S. Army

Master Sergeant Thomas A. Wallsmith died on October 26, 2005, when an improvised explosive device detonated near his vehicle in Rustamiyah, Iraq. In support of Operation Iraqi Freedom, the 38-year-old was assigned to the 3rd Forward Support Battalion, 3rd Infantry Division based in Fort Stewart, Georgia. Wallsmith's memorial service was held at the Pederson Funeral Home in Rockford, Michigan, after which the Soldier was buried in the Fort Custer National Cemetery in Augusta, Michigan.

Wallsmith entered the Army in 1987. He graduated from the Army's Respiratory Therapy Program in 1992, and served in that specialty role at Brooke Army Medical Center's Institute of Surgical Research in San Antonio, Texas. He also practiced as a Respiratory Therapist at William Beaumont Medical Center in El Paso, Texas, and Tripler Army Medical Center in Honolulu, Hawaii.

Thomas' survivors include his wife, Brenda; his daughter, Lauren; his son, Nathaniel; his parents, David and Carol; and his brother, Joel.

JEFFREY L. WIENER
Died: May 7, 2005
Branch: U.S. Navy

Petty Officer Third Class Jeffrey L. Wiener was killed during a firefight with insurgents on May 7, 2005, in western Iraq. The 32-year-old Hospital Corpsman was assigned to the 3rd Battalion, 25th Marine Regiment, 2nd Marine Division, II Marine Expeditionary Force. Grieving family and friends gathered on May 16, 2005, to bid their final farewells to their fallen husband, father, son, and brother at the Calverton National Cemetery in New York.

Jeff leaves behind to cherish his memory, his wife, Mariateresa; children, Mikayla Lynn and Theadora Rose; his parents, Diana and Wayne; his sisters, Wendi, Jessica, and Delayne; and his brothers Joshua and David.

JEFFREY A. WILLIAMS
Died: September 5, 2005
Branch: U.S. Army

Specialist Jeffrey A. Williams was killed on September 5, 2005, when a hidden bomb detonated near his combat vehicle in Tal Afar, Iraq, while he was serving in support of Operation Iraqi Freedom. Specialist Williams was a Combat Medic assigned to the Support Squadron, 3rd Armored Cavalry Regiment out of Fort Carson, Colorado.

He was buried in Fort Leavenworth National Cemetery, in Fort Leavenworth, Kansas. Williams went through basic training at Fort Benning, Georgia, and advanced individual training at Fort Sam Houston, Texas. While at Fort Carson in 2004, he took medical classes through a correspondence course at Texas Central University. He hoped to become a cardiologist, and had begun taking courses toward that goal. Williams came from a long military tradition. His mother worked as a civilian nurse at military hospitals, and several members of his family served in the military. During his weekly calls home to his mother, he would share stories of what medical procedures he had performed, including the time he inserted his first chest tube in a wounded patient.

Jeff is survived by his fiancée, Stacey Kuhn; his parents, Aron and Sandra; his brothers, Jermaine, Jerren, LeSean, CJ, Jalen, and Dennis; his sister, Madyson; and his grandparents, Tim and Eatha.

ERIC P. WOODS
Died: July 9, 2005
Branch: U.S. Army

Private First Class Eric P. Woods was killed July 9, 2005, when an improvised explosive device detonated near his vehicle outside Tal Afair, Iraq. Woods, who was assigned to the 2nd Squadron, 3rd Armored Cavalry Regiment out of Fort Carson, Colorado, died heroically while performing the duties of a Combat Medic, attempting to save a comrade's life. Shortly before the explosion, Woods had aided a wounded Soldier, stabilizing him and loading him onto a vehicle for transportation. As they drove to the landing zone, Woods' vehicle was struck by a bomb, which killed both Woods and another Soldier. The Soldier initially aided by Woods, Sergeant Wolfsteller, survived. Woods was buried with full military honors in McDivitt Grove Cemetery in Urbandale, Iowa.

While he was in Iraq, he asked his family to send toys, candy, and soccer balls for the Iraqi children. He also asked for items that would help other Soldiers, such as foot powder, moist towelettes, and lip balm. An avid reader of Stephen King novels, Woods also enjoyed crossword puzzles and playing Texas Hold 'Em poker with troopers of his platoon. Shortly before he died, Woods was offered a chance to move away from the front lines. He turned down that opportunity, believing he could do more to help his fellow Soldiers from where he was, he told his father the morning he died.

Woods' awards and decorations include the Bronze Star, Purple Heart, Good Conduct Medal, Army Commendation Medal, and Combat Medical Badge.

Eric is survived by his wife, Jamie, and son, Eric; his parents, Charles and Janis; and countless friends and fellow service members.

BENYAHMIN B. YAHUDAH
Died: July 13, 2005
Branch: U.S. Army

Specialist Benyahmin Yahudah was killed in a suicide bombing in Baghdad, Iraq, on July 13, 2005. He was trying to move children out of the area as Coalition Soldiers conducted a search. Sadly, 18 children died in the same incident. In his last moments, two of his Soldiers saw "DOC" bandaging one of the children. The 24-year-old was assigned to the 1st Battalion, 64th Armor Regiment, 2nd Brigade Combat Team, 3rd Infantry Division out of Fort Stewart, Georgia, supporting Operation Iraqi Freedom. Yahudah was laid to rest at Evergreen Memorial Park in Athens, Georgia.

On the day of Yahudah's death, Private First Class A. J. Arnett was lying wounded on the ground. Arnett is still overwhelmed with Doc's (as he was affectionately called) unbelievable passion for helping the children of Iraq. As Arnett lay wounded, he looked over at Doc, who was lying amongst the injured children. Arnett remembers seeing him put a bandage on a small child in his last moments. The last unconditional selfless act of a man who found joy among the smiling happy faces of children will live on in his memories of those who were lucky enough to have witnessed a simple act of kindness.

Benyahmin leaves behind his mother, Leah; siblings, Kirk, Elaine, Olga, Bethsheba, Shoshanah, Yahosuah, Ben; and his fiancée, Annie.

TRAVIS L. YOUNGBLOOD

Died: July 21, 2005
Branch: U.S. Navy

Petty Officer Third Class Travis L. Youngblood, a 26-year-old Navy Corpsman assigned to the Naval Hospital Great Lakes in Great Lakes, Illinois, lost his life on July 21, 2005, from wounds received on July 15, 2005. Youngblood was conducting combat operations in Hit, Iraq, when he was struck by shrapnel from an improvised explosive device. He was in Iraq fighting alongside and tending to the Marines of the 2nd Marine Division, II Marine Expeditionary Force supporting Operation Iraqi Freedom. Youngblood received a hero's burial when he was laid to rest in Arlington National Cemetery, Arlington, Virginia, on August 1, 2005, just eight weeks before the birth of his daughter.

Travis was born at Pensacola Naval Base in Florida on June 5, 1979. He was a member of the Southampton High School drama club in Courtland, Virginia, and graduated in 1997. In 1999 Travis married Laura, and in 2000, they had a son, Hunter. Tragically, Travis did not get to meet the child his wife was pregnant with at the time of his death.

Travis is survived by his wife, Laura; his children, Hunter and Emmy; and his parents Elmer and Debra.

DUSTIN M. ADKINS

Died: December 4, 2006
Branch: U.S. Army

Sergeant Dustin M. Adkins was killed on December 4, 2006, when the helicopter in which he was riding crashed near Haditha, Iraq, due to mechanical problems. On his second tour in Iraq, Adkins served as a Dental Assistant in support of Operation Iraqi Freedom with the Group Support Battalion, 5th Special Forces Group out of Fort Campbell, Kentucky. An exemplary Soldier, he was also a fully trained Special Forces Soldier. Adkins is buried in Cave Springs Cemetery in Henderson, Tennessee.

In Iraq, Adkins distinguished himself as the traveling Dental Technician. He often traveled in hazardous areas and endured austere living conditions in order to provide quality dental care to U.S. servicemembers and Iraqis.

Dustin leaves behind his wife, Tiffany; children, Matthew and Atlanta; his mother, Karen, and father Richard; and his brother and sister, Nicholas and Crystal.

NATHANIEL A. AGUIRRE
Died: October 22, 2006
Branch: U.S. Army

Corporal Nathaniel A. Aguirre was killed on October 22, 2006, by a sniper in Iraq. He was a Medic with Headquarters Company, 1st Battalion, 22nd Infantry Regiment, 1st Brigade Combat Team, 4th Infantry Division at Fort Hood, Texas. According to reports, Aguirre had run out into the open, exposing himself to enemy fire, to save a wounded fellow Soldier, most likely knowing that he would be the next person targeted in the ambush. In keeping with his dedication to his fellow Soldiers, Aguirre had volunteered for the mission because the unit involved did not have a Medic that day. He was 21 years old. He is buried in his hometown of Carrollton, Texas.

Aguirre could not wait to serve his country, and joined the Reserves while still in high school. He was not yet 18 years old, and so his mother, Mary, had to give special permission for him to join. Aguirre graduated from basic training at Fort Benning, Georgia, and advanced individual training at Fort Sam Houston, Texas, and then graduated from Army Airborne School at Fort Benning.

Nathaniel's devotion to his country was recognized by those in his hometown, where thousands of people lined the streets between the memorial service and his final resting place. Among them were Boy Scouts in uniform saluting the hearse as it passed. His military escort included a neighbor's son who had just returned from a tour in Iraq. Local businesses lowered their flags in his honor.

Nathaniel is survived by his parents, Louis and Mary.

ZACHARY M. ALDAY

Died: June 9, 2006
Branch: U.S. Navy

U.S. Navy Hospital Corpsman Zach M. Alday was killed while riding as a passenger in a Humvee on June 9, 2006, in Iraq. His vehicle struck a land mine as it was carrying out combat operations against enemy forces. Alday had been serving in Operation Iraqi Freedom with the 1st Battalion, 7th Marine Regiment, 1st Marine Division, I Marine Expeditionary Force based at Camp Pendleton, California. His relatives and friends grieved the 22-year-old Corpsman's passing at funeral services held June 19, 2006, at Spring Creek Baptist Church in Donalsonville, Georgia. Alday was buried in the church's cemetery. A United States Navy Honor Guard attended the burial as active pallbearers. Members of the local American Legion Post 157 were also present, serving in solemn tribute as honorary pallbearers.

Survivors include Zach's parents, Tommy and Donna; his daughter, Kamryn; his sister Mandy; and his grandparents.

DAVID J. ALMAZAN

Died: August 27, 2006
Branch: U.S. Army

Sergeant David Jimenez Almazan was killed on August 27, 2006, when an improvised explosive device detonated near his vehicle during combat operations in Hit, Iraq, while supporting Operation Iraqi Freedom. He was serving as a Combat Medic with the Army's 1st Battalion, 36th Infantry Regiment, 1st Brigade Combat Team, 1st Armored Division out of Germany. Almazan was buried at the Rose Hills Memorial Park in Whittier, California. He was awarded United States citizenship posthumously, effective the day of his death.

Born in Mexico, David had come to the United States when he was 11 years old. He never lost his appreciation for his Mexican heritage. He loved salsa dancing, and his favorite food was enchiladas with homemade rice, beans and Tapatio hot sauce. David always managed to see the good in people and never had one complaint. The way he spoke of his family and how much they meant to him made him a remarkable person.

Almazan is remembered as someone who always had time for others. He would take time out of his busy day to be there for others whether they needed someone to talk to, play cards with, or watch movies with.

In addition to his wife, Selena, David is survived by his parents, David and Olivia, and two sisters, Mayra and Mariana.

CHRISTOPHER A. ANDERSON
Died: December 4, 2006
Branch: U.S. Navy

Navy Petty Officer Third Class Chris A. Anderson died during an enemy mortar attack on December 4, 2006, near Ramadi, the capital of the Al Anbar Province in Iraq. The 24-year-old Corpsman was serving with the 1st Battalion, 6th Marine Regiment, 2nd Marine Division out of Camp Lejeune, North Carolina. His funeral took place on December 16, 2006, at the Grace Evangelical Free Church in his hometown of Longmont, Colorado.

A product of four generations of Navy men and women, Anderson joined the military in August 2005. He served his initial tour of duty with Longmont Navy Recruiting Office.

His father eulogized Chris as a "natural leader," who was "warm, giving, thoughtful and caring," adding that he was an encourager and an up lifter with a truly unique ability to empower others to rise to success.

Chris is survived by his parents Rick and Debra, and his brother Kyle.

RICHARD A. BLAKLEY
Died: June 6, 2006
Branch: U.S. Army

Staff Sergeant Richard A. Blakley was killed on June 6, 2006, by small-arms fire while patrolling the city of Al Khalidiyah, Iraq.

He was assigned to E Company, 38th Main Support Battalion of the Indiana Army National Guard. Blakley was also a veteran of Operation Desert Shield/Desert Storm, serving in various ports during that conflict. Blakley was buried on June 15, 2007, at Clayton Cemetery in Avon, Indiana. Both Indiana Governor Mitch Daniels and Indiana National Guard Adjutant General Major General Martin Umbarger were among the attendees at the funeral.

On January 16, 2006, Blakley was hit by a bullet that went through his body armor at the back of his neck and penetrated his shoulder. He managed to get out of the line of fire, find cover, and radio for help. When treated in Iraq for that wound, he declined an opportunity to return home for full treatment. A dedicated Soldier and Medic, Blakley also refused an offer for a few days of rest and relaxation, and returned to his unit that same afternoon. He continued to treat his wound himself. When asked why, he explained that his men needed him.

Richard leaves behind his wife, Patty, and their two children, Whitney and Rick.

JEFFREY S. BROWN
Died: August 8, 2006
Branch: U.S. Army

Sergeant Jeffrey S. Brown was killed on August 8, 2006, when the helicopter in which he was riding crashed into a lake in Rutbah, Iraq, while supporting Operation Iraqi Freedom. The 25-year-old Crew Chief served with the 82nd Medical Company out of Fort Riley, Kansas. Sergeant Steven Mennemeyer, a Medic, also died in the crash. Brown was cremated and his ashes scattered on his family's land.

Jeff is survived by his wife, Ashley; parents, Ed and Diane; his brothers, Michael and Timothy; and his sister, Kathryn.

HEATHE N. CRAIG
Died: June 21, 2006
Branch: U.S. Army

Staff Sergeant Heathe N. Craig died on June 21, 2006, when his helicopter hoist malfunctioned in Naray, Afghanistan, where he was serving in support of Operation Enduring Freedom. While attempting to evacuate another Soldier hurt during combat operations, Craig was holding the wounded Soldier as they were both hoisted from a ridgeline by the helicopter. Halfway to the helicopter, the line snapped and both Soldiers fell to their deaths. The 28-year-old was assigned to the 159th Medical Company out of Wiesbaden, Germany. Craig's memorial service and funeral were held at Wiesbaden Army Airfield's Chapel.

Craig wanted to help people. He even considered becoming a kindergarten teacher until the desire to join the Army intervened. There, he learned his true calling was as a Combat Medic.

Heathe is survived by his wife Judith; his son Jonas, and his daughter Leona; as well as his father Jeffrey and his mother, Donna.

DAVID N. CROMBIE
Died: June 7, 2006
Branch: U.S. Army

Private First Class David N. Crombie died on June 7, 2006, when an improvised explosive device detonated near his vehicle in Iraq. He was assigned to the 2nd Battalion, 6th Infantry Regiment out of Baumholder, Germany. At the time of his death, he was attached to Task Force 1-35 of the 1st Armored Division, serving with the I Marine Expeditionary Force. That group was one of the first military units to go into unsettled areas of Iraq in support of Operation Iraqi Freedom, where the risk of IEDs was extremely high. Crombie was buried with full military honors at Arlington, Virginia.

Crombie was determined to join the Army despite his asthma. Faced with initial rejection after an asthma attack, he refused to allow the Army to deny him his chance, and joined in 2005. He successfully finished basic training at Fort Benning, and then trained as a Medic at Fort Sam Houston, Texas.

David leaves behind his mother, Jennifer; brothers Dan and Jason; and his grandmother, Mary.

JASON B. DANIEL
Died: April 23, 2006
Branch: U.S. Army

Corporal Jason B. Daniel died April 23, 2006, in Taji, Iraq, when an improvised explosive device detonated near his Humvee during combat operations. The 21-year-old Medic was assigned to the 7th Squadron, 10th Cavalry Regiment, 1st Brigade Combat Team, 4th Infantry Division out of Fort Hood, Texas. Two other Soldiers died in the same incident. Daniel was buried with full military honors at the Fort Sam Houston National Cemetery in Texas.

Jason's fellow Soldiers recall their fallen comrade's smile and happy attitude. The Griffin family, of Fort Hood, Texas, welcomed Daniel into their extended family where he would join them for cookouts. They remember him as an honest, friendly guy, who had a smile for everyone and always wanted to help others if he could.

Jason leaves behind his wife, Monika; mother Linda; father Henry; sister, Teagan; and grandparents, John and Margaret.

DAVID J. DAVIS
Died: September 17, 2006
Branch: U.S. Army

Sergeant David J. Davis lost his life on September 17, 2006, when an improvised explosive device (IED) detonated near the vehicle in which he was riding, near Sadr City, Iraq. Two other Soldiers in the vehicle were also wounded. Davis was 32 years old and served with the 4th Squadron, 14th Cavalry Regiment, 172nd Stryker Brigade Combat Team out of Fort Wainwright, Alaska. Davis joined the Army in April 2003, and trained as a Medic. Davis was buried in Polar Springs Cemetery in Mount Airy, Maryland, on September 28, 2006.

David leaves behind his wife, Bobbie; his parents Jim and Josephine; his brother, James; and his sisters, Theresa and Helen.

LEE H. DEAL

Died: May 17, 2006
Branch: U.S. Navy

Petty Officer Third Class Lee H. Deal died May 17, 2006, as a result of injuries sustained in combat while clearing a suspected insurgent stronghold in Anbar Province, Iraq. He was assigned to the 2nd Reconnaissance Battalion, 5th Marine Regiment, 2nd Marine Division out of Camp Lejeune, North Carolina. Deal is buried at the Roselawn Memorial Garden in Calhoun, Louisiana.

Lee is survived by his father, Harry; his mother, Melanie; his brother, Justin; and his fiancée, Margaret.

ADAM L. FARGO

Died: July 22, 2006
Branch: U.S. Army

Corporal Adam L. Fargo lost his life on July 22, 2006, while his unit was conducting convoy operations in Baghdad, Iraq. The vehicle Fargo was driving was attacked by small-arms fire, and an improvised explosive device (IED) detonated within two meters of the vehicle on the driver's side, killing Fargo immediately. Four other Soldiers were wounded in the blast. Fargo was assigned to Headquarters Company, 4th Brigade Troop Battalion, 4th Brigade Combat Team, 101st Airborne Division in support of Operation Iraqi Freedom. Fargo was buried with full military honors in Culpeper National Cemetery, Culpeper, Virginia, on July 31, 2006.

Fargo is survived by his parents, Douglas and Elizabeth; his brother, Jason; and his sister, Sarah.

JOHN T. FRALISH, II
Died: February 6, 2006
Branch: U.S. Navy

Petty Officer Third Class John T. Fralish, II, died from chest wounds incurred when enemy forces fired on his patrol northwest of Methar Lam, Afghanistan, on February 6, 2006. He was serving as a Hospital Corpsman for the 1st Battalion, 3rd Marine Regiment supporting Operation Enduring Freedom. The 30-year-old Sailor was garrisoned at the Marine Corps Base Hawaii. On February 18, 2006, his funeral services took place at the Hoffman-Roth Funeral Home and his burial followed at the Cumberland Valley Memorial Gardens in Carlisle, Pennsylvania.

Inspired by the 9/11 terrorist attacks, his father's Navy Reserve service in Vietnam, and his grandfather, Army Colonel John C. Fralish, a WWII and Korean War veteran, Fralish enlisted in the Navy in February 2002.

John is survived by his parents, James and Jean; three brothers and two sisters; his fiancée, Cynthia; and his grandparents.

ANTHONY R. GARCIA
Died: February 17, 2006
Branch: U.S. Army

Army Captain Anthony Garcia died from a gunshot wound on February 17, 2006, on an Army base in Tikrit, Iraq. Garcia was a Physician Assistant with the Headquarters Company, 1st Battalion, 101st Aviation Regiment, 101st Airborne Division. Garcia was buried with full military honors in Dallas National Cemetery in Texas.

Garcia enlisted in the Army in 1989, at age 32. He served in Operation Desert Shield/Desert Storm, then in a variety of units before graduating from the University of Texas at Austin and becoming a Physician Assistant. He had served in Afghanistan and had a previous tour of duty in Iraq.

Anthony is survived by his wife, Doris; his daughter, Kelly, and his son, Garrick.

DANIEL R. GIONET
Died: June 4, 2006
Branch: U.S. Army

Sergeant Daniel R. Gionet was killed June 4, 2006, when the tank he was riding in hit an explosive device near Taji, Iraq. The 24-year-old had been serving as the Medic with the 1st Battalion, 66th Armor Regiment, 1st Brigade Combat Team, 4th Infantry Division out of Fort Hood, Texas. After being wounded, he tended to those around him. When medical units arrived, Gionet, apparently unconcerned with the severity of his own wounds, directed them to treat others first. "Don't deal with me," he said, moments before dying. Gionet was buried with full military honors at Gibson Cemetery in Massachusetts, just across the state line from his hometown of Pelham, New Hampshire.

Daniel leaves behind his wife, Katrina; his mother, Denise; father, Daniel; brother and sister, Darren and Alycia; and his grandparents.

AARON M. GRINER
Died: June 28, 2006
Branch: U.S. Army

Corporal Aaron M. Griner died on June 28, 2006, in the Helmand Province of Afghanistan when his vehicle struck a land mine while supporting Operation Enduring Freedom. He was assigned to HQ Company, 2nd Battalion, 87th Infantry Regiment, 3rd Brigade Combat Team, 10th Mountain Division out of Fort Drum, New York. A funeral mass was given on Friday, July 14, 2006, at Sacred Heart Catholic Church in Tampa, Florida.

When he joined the Army, Aaron was seeking a career; what he found was a young woman named Amanda who became his wife. Aaron's son, Austin, was born only a few weeks before his unit deployed. The Army delayed his actual deployment until Austin was a month old, giving the young family a little more time together.

He is survived by his wife, Amanda, and his son, Austin; his mother and father, Anita and Ernest; sisters Annie and Megan; and a large extended family.

RICHARD J. HERREMA
Died: April 25, 2006
Branch: U.S. Army

Sergeant First Class Richard J. Herrema died on April 25, 2006, from wounds received during combat operations in Baghdad, Iraq. The 27-year-old Soldier's unit had received intelligence concerning some insurgent activity and, in response, mounted an attack on the enemy. Herrema was the first man off his helicopter, and the enemy fire hit him almost instantly. Although he was evacuated to a nearby field hospital, his wounds were fatal. His family buried him in Forest Grove Cemetery in Jamestown, Michigan.

He is survived by his parents, Richard and Mary; and his sisters, Katie Lynn and Janie Lynn.

ANTON J. HIETT
Died: March 12, 2006
Branch: U.S. Army

Sergeant Anton J. Hiett died on March 12, 2006, when an IED detonated near his patrol in Afghanistan. Three other Soldiers died in the same incident. Hiett was 25 years old and serving with the 391st Engineer Battalion, U.S. Army Reserve out of North Carolina. He had recently transferred to that unit when he learned that his own unit would not deploy to either Iraq or Afghanistan. The unit had arrived in that part of Afghanistan only a couple days earlier. The Army Honor Guard of Fort Bragg gave full military honors at Sergeant Hiett's burial in the Salisbury National Cemetery, Salisbury, North Carolina, on March 25, 2006.

George Hiett, a Vietnam veteran, said he supported his son's decision to go to Afghanistan. The two had talked about the risks, and Anton knew that it was not going to be easy. "You know, we live in a free country, but no one wants their child to die," his father said. "I also know that someone has to fight the battle, and freedom has a price."

Anton is survived by his wife, Misty; his daughter, Kyra; his parents, George and Angela; two brothers, Tyrone and Immanuel; and sister, Sonia.

MERIDETH L. HOWARD
Died: September 8, 2006
Branch: U.S. Army

Sergeant First Class Merideth L. Howard died September 8, 2006, in Kabul, Afghanistan, when a car bomb exploded near the Humvee in which she was riding as the gunner. At 52 years old, she was the oldest American woman to die in combat in U.S. history. She was assigned to the 364th Civil Affairs Brigade in support of the 10th Mountain Division, acting as a liaison between the Afgan people and the military in support of Operation Enduring Freedom. Her husband scattered her ashes in two firework displays.

Merideth is survived by her husband, Hugh.

MATTHEW D. HUNTER
Died: January 23, 2006
Branch: U.S. Army

Sergeant Matthew D. Hunter was killed in Baghdad, Iraq, on January 23, 2006, when an improvised explosive device detonated near his dismounted patrol during combat operations. He was assigned to the 1st Battalion, 502nd Infantry Regiment, 2nd Brigade Combat Team, 101st Airborne Division out of Fort Campbell, Kentucky, in support of Operation Iraqi Freedom. Matthew was laid to rest in West Alexander Cemetery in Pennsylvania.

Matt was a native of Valley Grove, West Virginia. High school classmates from Wheeling Park High School in nearby Wheeling, West Virginia, recalled that Matt always wanted to enter the Army. He followed his dream, entering the military in 1995. He was so proud of being a Soldier that he wore his dress uniform to his 10-year high school reunion in 2002.

Soldiers said Hunter was living his dream in a world where so many are not. They remember the simple things he did, like helping relieve simple aches and pains, and his great taste in music. He cared deeply and had strong values.

Matt is survived by his wife, Wendy; his mother and father Kathy and Fred; and a brother and sister.

WAKKUNA A. JACKSON
Died: August 19, 2006
Branch: U.S. Army

Sergeant Wakkuna Jackson died in Kunar Province, Afghanistan, on August 19, 2006, when an improvised explosive device detonated near her convoy, which was then attacked by Taliban fighters. The convoy was delivering supplies to a hospital serving women and children. Sergeant Jackson was assigned to the 710th Combat Support Battalion, 3rd Brigade Combat Team, 10th Mountain Division out of Fort Drum, New York, in support of Operation Enduring Freedom. She was buried in Edgewood Cemetery near Jacksonville, Florida, on September 1, 2006. She was 21. Wakkuna's desire to help people predated her service as a Medic. A compassionate child, she always reached out to others. At age 17, she cut off her hair and donated it to a local cancer society. Family noted that this was just one example of her empathetic nature.

Wakkuna is survived by her parents, Sherman and Teresita, and two sisters.

JAMIE S. JAENKE
Died: June 5, 2006
Branch: U.S. Navy

Petty Officer Second Class Jamie S. Jaenke, a Navy Reservist assigned to Naval Mobile Construction Battalion out of Fort McCoy, Wisconsin, lost her life on June 5, 2006, while serving her country in

Iraq, when the vehicle she was riding in was struck by an IED. The 29-year-old Seabee, the third Navy female to die in Iraq, had been serving as a Paramedic in support of Operation Iraqi Freedom for less than three months. Her funeral services were held June 14, 2006, at the First United Methodist Church in Iowa Falls, Iowa.

Jamie leaves behind her 9-year-old daughter, Kayla.

CHARLES J. JONES
Died: September 20, 2006
Branch: U.S. Army

Sergeant First Class Charles J. Jones died in Camp Liberty, Iraq, on September 20, 2006, while supporting Operation Iraqi Freedom. The 29-year-old Medic was assigned to the 149th Brigade Combat Team, which is commanded by his father, Colonel Charles T. Jones. Colonel Jones was serving in Tikrit, Iraq, at the time of his son's death. Kentucky Governor Ernie Fletcher ordered flags in the state to be flown at half-staff in the days leading up to Jones' funeral. He was buried in Locust Grove Cemetery in Keavy, Kentucky.

Charles is survived by his parents, Colonel Charles and Linda Jones; and sister, Brandi.

DALE J. KELLY, JR.
Died: May 6, 2006
Branch: U.S. Army

Staff Sergeant Dale Kelly, Jr., dreamed of providing a full barbeque feast for his fellow Soldiers in Iraq. Fate denied him that opportunity, however, when an improvised explosive device hit his vehicle during combat operations in Iraq on May 6, 2006. Kelly was serving in support of Operation Iraqi Freedom with the Army National Guard's 3rd Battalion, 172nd Infantry Regiment out of Brewer, Maine. The unit was deployed to provide security operations for convoys in Iraq. Kelly was riding in the lead vehicle at the time of the attack, serving as a Medic. Kelly was buried with full military honors at the Maine Veteran's Memorial Cemetery in Augusta, Maine.

Dale is survived by his wife, Nancy, and three children, Julie, Christopher, and Jennifer.

CHADWICK T. KENYON
Died: August 20, 2006
Branch: U.S. Navy

Navy Hospital Corpsman Chadwick T. Kenyon was assigned to the 3rd Light Armored Reconnaissance Battalion, 1st Marine Division out of Twentynine Palms, California, when he died on August 20, 2006. The 20-year-old was conducting combat operations against enemy forces in the Al Anbar Province, Iraq, when the vehicle he was riding in was struck by an improvised explosive device. Family and friends said their final farewells at the Evergreen Mortuary Cemetery in Tucson, Arizona.

Chad is survived by his parents, Charmaine and Douglas.

JANE E. LANHAM
Died: September 19, 2006
Branch: U.S. Navy

Lieutenant Commander Jane E. Lanham died unexpectedly of natural causes on September 19, 2006, while in Manama, Bahrain, in support of Operation Iraqi Freedom. The 43-year-old Sailor was assigned to the Naval Branch Health Clinic in Manama. She is buried in Resurrection Cemetery in Daviess County, Kentucky.

Jane is survived by her husband John, and daughters, Rachel and Natalie.

JEREMY LOVELESS
Died: May 29, 2006
Branch: U.S. Army

Corporal Jeremy Loveless was killed by a sniper during combat operations on May 29, 2006, in Mosul, Iraq. While serving as a lookout, outside the protection of his Stryker vehicle, Loveless was shot in the shoulder unbeknownst to fellow Soldiers. The 25-year-old was assigned to the medical platoon of the 2nd Battalion, 1st Infantry Regiment, 172nd Stryker Brigade Combat Team out of Fort Wainwright, Alaska, in support of Operation Iraqi Freedom. Loveless was laid to rest with full military honors at George Cemetery in Estacada, Oregon.

Jeremy leaves behind his wife, Meredith, and daughter, Chloe.

THOMAS D. MAHOLIC
Died: June 24, 2006
Branch: U.S. Army

Master Sergeant Thomas D. Maholic lost his life on June 24, 2006, while supporting his country in Operation Enduring Freedom. The 38-year-old Green Beret was conducting a cordon and search mission in Ghecko, Afghanistan, when his patrol unit came under fire from enemy forces. A 17-hour battle ensued, and he was hit by small-arms fire. Master Sergeant Maholic was assigned as a Medical Sergeant to the 2nd Battalion, 7th Special Forces Group based at Fort Bragg, North Carolina. He is buried at Willow Dale Cemetery in Bradford, Pennsylvania.

A fellow Soldier wrote to Tom's family, "I had the honor of meeting Tom and seeing him and his team work a couple of months ago outside Kandahar. It was obvious that he was truly a quiet professional. I cannot speak more highly of a warrior. Thank you for giving us such a fine American and fine Soldier, he will be missed."

Tom is survived by his wife, Wendy; his son, Andrew; his mother, Dorothy; a sister, Ann; brothers, David, John, Michael and Robert; and numerous family and friends.

STEVEN P. MENNEMEYER
Died: August 8, 2006
Branch: U.S. Army

Sergeant Steven P. Mennemeyer died on August 8, 2006, in Anbar Province, Iraq. On his second tour in Iraq, Mennemeyer was serving as a Flight Medic assigned to the 82nd Medical Company out of Fort Riley, Kansas. Sergeant Mennemeyer died when his helicopter crashed into a lake in the vicinity of Rutbah, Iraq. Also killed was Sergeant Jeffrey S. Brown. Family and friends gathered for a memorial service and celebration of his life in Granite City, Illinois. He was buried with full military honors in the Jefferson Barracks National Cemetery, St. Louis, Missouri.

Steven is survived by his mother, Ramona; his father, Steve; his son, Andrew; sister Sarah, and many friends and extended family.

MARCQUES J. NETTLES
Died: April 2, 2006
Branch: U.S. Navy

Petty Officer Third Class Marcques J. Nettles was killed April 2, 2006, in Anbar Province, Iraq, when the truck he was riding in during a combat logistics convoy rolled over in a flash flood. The 22-year-old Corpsman had been in Iraq for less than three months at the time of his death. A remembrance of Nettles' life was held on May 7, 2006, at the New Beginnings Christian Center in Portland, Oregon.

Motivated by a desire to pursue a nursing career, and following in the footsteps of his big brother, Curtis, he enlisted in the Navy on September 11, 2002, and was assigned to Force Service Regiment, Fleet Marine Forces Pacific. His career took him to Whidbey Island Naval Hospital, Washington. He deployed to Iraq on February 14, 2006, in support of Operation Iraqi Freedom.

Marcques is survived by his wife, Christina; his parents, Curtis and Susan; his brother, Curtis Jr.; and his sisters Bianca and Manny.

KYLE A. NOLEN
Died: December 21, 2006
Branch: U.S. Navy

On December 21, 2006, 21-year-old Hospital Corpsman Kyle A. Nolen died as a result of injuries he received in a land mine explosion in Anbar Province, Iraq. The Ennis, Texas, native was assigned to the 3rd Battalion, 4th Marine Regiment, 1st Marine Division out of Twentynine Palms, California. Nolen was carried by horse-drawn carriage to his final resting spot in Myrtle Cemetery in Ennis. Nolen volunteered for the Navy in August 2005, fulfilling a boyhood pact he made with friends in elementary school to join the military. He became a Hospital Corpsman and received his assignment to Twentynine Palms in April 2006. He deployed for Iraq in August 2006 and had served less than four months at the time of his death.

Nolen is survived by his wife, Cassie and his children, Ryan and Railey; his parents Michael and Francis; his sisters, Angelica, Mikayla, Tori, and Sarah; and his brother, Shea.

GEOVANI PADILLA ALEMAN
Died: April 2, 2006
Branch: U.S. Navy

Hospital Corpsman Geovani Padilla Aleman, a Navy Hospital Corpsman, assigned to the National Naval Medical Center in Bethesda, Maryland, was killed on April 2, 2006, when a bomb exploded near the Humvee he was riding in while on patrol in Al Anbar Province west of Baghdad, Iraq. The 20-year-old was in Iraq with the United States Naval Service Comfort Detachment, providing medical care to the Marines of the 3rd Battalion, 8th Marine Regiment. Padilla Aleman had been in Iraq for only a month at the time of his death. Family and friends said their final farewells on April 14, 2006, at Rose Hill Memorial Chapel in Whittier, California, and he was buried at Rose Hill Memorial Park.

Geovani wrote his friend Nairoby Alvarez a letter shortly before his death in which he said, "We should not grieve when a hero dies. Instead, we should be grateful that he lived and consider ourselves privileged to have walked along his footsteps, if only for a short while."

He is survived by his proud family that includes his parents, a young sister, and many extended family members.

ROGER P. PENA, JR.

Died: June 14, 2006
Branch: U.S. Army

 Sergeant Roger P. Pena, Jr., lost his life while supporting his country in Operation Enduring Freedom. He died June 14, 2006, while on a resupply mission. The convoy he was in came under enemy small-arms fire during combat operations in Musa Qulah, Afghanistan. The 29-year-old Combat Medic had only recently been promoted to Sergeant. Sergeant Pena was assigned to the 10th Sustainment Brigade, 10th Mountain Division out of Fort Drum, New York. Funeral services for the fallen Soldier were held June 23, 2006, at the San Fernando Cathedral in San Antonio, Texas. He was laid in his final resting place with full military honors in Fort Sam Houston National Cemetery.

 Roger is survived by his wife, Marisol; his two sons, Ivan and Gabriel; his parents, Roger, Sr., and Paulita; his sisters, Karen, Yvette, and Annette; and his brother, Frederick.

JOHNNY J. PERALEZ, JR.

Died: January 5, 2006
Branch: U.S. Army

 Sergeant Johnny J. Peralez, Jr., lost his life on January 5, 2006, when an improvised explosive device detonated near the Humvee he was riding in while providing medical coverage during convoy operations in Iraq. The 25-year-old Soldier died while serving his second tour in support of Operation Iraqi Freedom. Sergeant Peralez was a medic for the 3rd Battalion, 16th Field Artillery Regiment, 2nd Brigade Combat Team, 4th Infantry Division out of Fort Hood, Texas. Family and friends gathered at the Sacred Heart Catholic Church in Falfurrias, Texas, on January 17, 2006, to say their final farewells to their hero before he was laid to rest at the Falfurrias Burial Park.

 Johnny's commander remembered him as a great professional, always ready for the unexpected. He trained the Medics under him to meet the same high standards.

Johnny is survived by his mother, Virginia; his father, Johnny; his sister, Nina; and his brothers, Romeo and Jessie.

EMILY JAZMIN TATUM PEREZ
Died: September 12, 2006
Branch: U.S. Army

Second Lieutenant Emily Jazmin Tatum Perez, from the 204th Support Battalion, 2nd Brigade Combat Team, 4th Infantry Division, was killed on September 12, 2006, when an improvised explosive device exploded under her Humvee as she was leading a convoy near Najaf in southern Iraq. Lieutenant Perez, from Fort Washington, Maryland, was 23 years old and was the first female graduate of West Point to die in Iraq. She is buried at the West Point Cemetery.

Emily, who had her choice of many universities, chose West Point for its academic and physical challenges, graduating in 2005 in the top 10 percent of her class. At West Point, she ran track, sang in the gospel choir, and helped start a dance squad to cheer for the football and basketball teams. She was the first minority female Command Sergeant Major of the Corps of Cadets in West Point history.

Emily is survived by her parents, Daniel and Vicki; a brother, Kevyn; and her grandparents.

DAVID J. RAMSEY
Died: September 7, 2006
Branch: U.S. Army

Specialist David J. Ramsey was medically evacuated from Mosul, Iraq, on August 24, 2006, as a result of a non-combat related incident. He died on September 7, 2006, in Spanaway, Washington. The 27-year-old Combat Medic was assigned to the 47th Combat Support Hospital, 62nd Medical Brigade out of Fort Lewis, Washington. Ramsey deployed to Iraq in support of Operation Iraqi Freedom in October 2005, proudly serving the 47th CSH in Mosul, Iraq. Friends and family said their final farewells on September 13, 2006, at the

Mountain View Funeral Home in Tacoma, Washington, before laying him to rest in Mountain View Memorial Park.

Davis is survived by his wife, Genesa; his parents, Joseph and Tok; and his sister, Christina.

NICHOLAS K. ROGERS
Died: October 22, 2006
Branch: U.S. Army

Specialist Nicholas K. Rogers died October 22, 2006, when his convoy was ambushed in Baghdad, Iraq. While under heavy small-arms and rocket fire, Specialist Rogers moved to his M240B machine gun and began suppressive fire. His actions allowed the pinned-down members of his platoon to move into position, achieving fire superiority, and suppress the enemy attack. Rogers served as a Combat Medic with the 4th Battalion, 31st Infantry Regiment, 2nd Brigade Combat Team, 10th Mountain Division out of Fort Drum, New York, in support of Operation Iraqi Freedom. He was buried with full military honors at Deltona Memorial Gardens in Deltona, Florida.

Nick is survived by his wife, Kelly; his daughters, Jocelyn and Isabelle; parents, Robert and Penny; and sister, Crystal.

CHARLES O. SARE
Died: October 23, 2006
Branch: U.S. Navy

United States Navy Hospital Corpsman Charles O. Sare perished on October 23, 2006, while serving in the Al Anbar Province, Iraq, in support of Operation Iraqi Freedom. His death resulted from injuries he sustained when an IED hit the vehicle in which he was a passenger. A final visitation took place on November 1, 2006, at Hemet's Miller-Jones Mortuary. Charles' funeral was held the next day at the Church of Jesus Christ of Latterday Saints in Hemet. Over 600 mourners attended the service, and Charles' favorite Toyota pickup truck took the lead in the procession of vehicles carrying his family and friends. Many of Sare's fellow Sailors have fond memories of going through boot camp and school with him. They recall that he was always ready with a laugh and a positive attitude about life. He was proud to serve his country and passed this enthusiasm on to his fellow comrades. Sare had a calling, and he answered it; he had a duty to perform, and he fulfilled it.

Surviving Charles are his parents, Charles and Karen; brother, Matt; and many friends and fellow Sailors.

CHRISTOPHER F. SITTON
Died: August 19, 2006
Branch: U.S. Army

Corporal Christopher F. Sitton was killed August 19, 2006, when an improvised explosive device detonated near his convoy, which was then attacked by Taliban fighters. The convoy was passing near the border with Pakistan en route to deliver supplies to a hospital from Camp Blessing in Kunar, Afghanistan, while supporting Operation Enduring Freedom. Two other Soldiers, one fellow Medic, died alongside the 21-year-old Sitton. Sitton served as Combat Medic with C Company, 710th Combat Support Battalion, 3rd Brigade Combat Team, 10th Mountain Division out of Fort Drum, New York. He was buried with full military honors in the Grand View Cemetery just outside Montrose, Texas.

Staff Sergeant Yvette Onwudiwe, a fellow Soldier who served with him at Fort Drum, thanked Sitton's parents for raising their son to be the man he was. "He knew how to be a friend to all, a person you turned to when there was no one else," she said, asking them to be proud of all he did, big and small. Sitton will always be remembered by those who loved him, including his C Company family who called out, "Thank you for all that you have done and all that you were to us."

Chris is survived by his parents, Steve and Judy; a sister, Laura; and his grandparents.

JOHN T. STONE
Died: March 28, 2006
Branch: U.S. Army

Sergeant First Class John T. Stone was killed by enemy mortar and small-arms attacks during combat operations in Lashkagar, Afghanistan, on March 28, 2006. He was shot several times while supporting Afghan Army Soldiers his unit was helping to train. The 52-year-old Soldier was assigned to the 15th Civil Support Team, Vermont National Guard out of South Burlington, Vermont. He was on his third tour in Afghanistan, supporting Operation Enduring Freedom. He is buried in Saint Anthony Cemetery in Wilder, Vermont.

In Afghanistan, Stone set up public medical clinics near forward operating bases to treat local civilians. He was credited with saving hundreds of Afghan lives. Fellow Soldiers remember Stone as a well-respected, compassionate role model, dedicated to caring for those around him.

John is survived by his life partner, Rose, and his sister, Roberta.

DOUGLAS L. TINSLEY
Died: December 26, 2006
Branch: U.S. Army

Specialist Douglas L. Tinsley died December 26, 2006, of injuries sustained when the vehicle in which he was riding rolled over into a canal in Baghdad, Iraq. The 21-year-old Soldier was conducting a mounted patrol at the time. Another Soldier died in the same incident, and a third was seriously injured. Specialist Tinsley was assigned to D Company, 3rd Battalion, 509th Parachute Infantry Regiment, 4th Brigade Combat Team, 25th Infantry Division out of Fort Richardson, Alaska, to support Operation Iraqi Freedom. He was buried with full military honors at Chester Memorial Gardens, South Carolina, on January 6, 2007.

Specialist Brooke Robson trained with Tinsley at Fort Sam Houston and fondly recalls how he had such an upbeat and wonderful personality. For Robson and many others, the world is a sadder place without him.

Douglas is survived by his mother, Lori; his father, Douglas; brother Private First Class Ryan Tinsley; sister, Kristen; and fiancée, Sarah.

ANGELO J. VACCARO
Died: October 2, 2006
Branch: U.S. Army

Corporal Angelo Joseph Vaccaro died on October 2, 2006, in Korengal, Afghanistan, while rescuing fellow Soldiers during combat operations in support of Operation Enduring Freedom. Vaccaro was a Medic with the 1st Battalion, 32nd Infantry Regiment, 3rd Brigade Combat Team, 10th Mountain Division out of Fort Drum, New York. Upon discovering that two of his platoon's Soldiers had been injured in a firefight, Vaccaro set out to retrieve the men. Reaching the most seriously wounded Soldier, Vaccaro shielded him with his own body, returned fire to the enemy, and then dragged the wounded trooper to a secure area. While returning to recover another Soldier, however, Vaccaro was killed by a rocket attack. On October 14, 2006, Vaccaro was buried at the Deltona Memorial Gardens in Orange City, Florida.

Corporal Angelo Vaccaro received a number of awards that illustrate the caliber of his service and commemorate his heroism: two Silver Stars, the Purple Heart, Army Achievement Medal, and the Combat Medic Badge. The 10th Mountain Division dedicated its Medical Simulation Training Center at Fort Drum to Angelo and another valiant medic who distinguished himself during WWII, Horace A. Bridgewater. The center became known as the Bridgewater-Vaccaro Center. Additionally, the HQ building of the Warrior Transition Brigade at Walter Reed Army Medical Center was renamed Vaccaro Hall.

Angelo is survived by his wife, Dana; his parents, Ray and Linda; his brothers, Vincent and Ray; and his sister, Christina.

NATHAN J. VACHO
Died: May 5, 2006
Branch: U.S. Army

Staff Sergeant Nathan J. Vacho was killed on May 5, 2006, when an improvised explosive device detonated near his Humvee during combat operations in Baghdad, Iraq. Two other Soldiers died in the same incident. The 29-year-old Kentucky Reservist had been in Iraq only two weeks as part of a mission to rebuild Iraqi villages. He had volunteered to deploy to Iraq as a Combat Medic with a Civil Affairs Battalion based in Tennessee. On the day of his funeral, both sides of Highway 8 near the Ladysmith High School in Ladysmith, Wisconsin, were lined with Patriot Guard members and their bikes. Many had come from other states to show their support for his family. Vacho was buried at Riverside Cemetery in Ladysmith.

Sergeant Charles Lovelace recalls that Vacho "was one of the best Soldiers I've ever worked with." Vacho's commander, Major Geraldine Kass, said, "He was a Soldier who had so much enthusiasm and was so positive."

Nathan is survived by his wife, Amanda; his daughters Emma Grace and Bayli; his father and mother, John and Carol; and his sister, Ashley.

RUBEN J. VILLA, JR.
Died: August 18, 2006
Branch: U.S. Army

Sergeant First Class Ruben J. Villa, Jr., died on August 18, 2006, in Dubai, United Arab Emirates, from a non-combat related cause. He was assigned to the Area Support Group, Coalition Forces Land Component Command out of Camp Arifjan in Kuwait. He was laid to rest at Fort Bliss National Cemetery in El Paso, Texas, on August 30, 2006.

Ruben is survived by his wife, Cecilia; daughters, Kristle, April, and Jacqui; and son, Raul.

RYAN D. WALKER
Died: January 5, 2006
Branch: U.S. Army

Specialist Ryan D. Walker was killed on January 5, 2006, when an improvised explosive device (IED) detonated near his Humvee in Baghdad, Iraq. During convoy operations supporting Operation Iraqi Freedom, the 25-year-old Medic was trying to help Soldiers injured by an IED when a second IED detonated near him. Another Soldier was killed in the same incident. Walker was assigned to the 1st Battalion, 76th Field Artillery Regiment, 4th Brigade Combat Team, 3rd Infantry Division out of Fort Stewart, Georgia. Family and friends buried Ryan on January 16, 2006, in Pilot Rock Cemetery in Pilot Rock, Oregon.

Specialist Walker was posthumously awarded two Bronze Stars for valor and a Purple Heart, in addition to two Purple Hearts awarded to him before his death.

Ryan is survived by his father, Randall; his mother, Louise; and his brother, Steven.

CHRISTOPHER G. WALSH
Died: September 4, 2006
Branch: U.S. Navy

Petty Officer Second Class Chris G. Walsh, a Navy Reserve Hospital Corpsman, heroically gave his life while serving his country on September 4, 2006. Walsh was conducting combat operations in Al Anbar Province, Iraq, when his vehicle was struck by a roadside bomb. The 30-year-old Corpsman was assigned to the 3rd Battalion, 24th Marine Regiment, 4th Marine Division out of Bridgeton, Missouri. After an escort back to the United States by his brother, a Marine, funeral services were held for Walsh September 15, 2006, at St. Joseph Catholic Church, followed by his burial in Fort Leavenworth National Cemetery.

Driven by a passion to save lives and following in the footsteps of his father, a Medic who served in Vietnam, Walsh volunteered for the Navy Reserves and trained as a Corpsman, with his first assignment in Fallujah, Iraq, in March 2006.

Walsh's good deeds went beyond his service to his country. They stretched across cultural boundaries when he went beyond the call of duty to tend to the needs of an Iraqi baby in desperate need of an operation. While on patrol searching for a sniper, Walsh and his unit were approached by a desperate mother with a visibly sick baby. Walsh put down his gun and examined the baby, taking pictures to show the Chief Medical Officer, convincing him that they needed to help that baby. After an incredible amount of red tape, the baby, Mariam, was wheeled into the operating room at Massachusetts General on October 13, a month and a half after Walsh's death. She came through the surgery just fine. Mariam's grandfather asked Walsh's mother, who flew to Boston, to meet the child her son fought so hard to save.

Chris is survived by his mother, Maureen; brothers, Patrick and Joseph; and sisters, Erin and Meghan.

JAMES R. WORSTER
Died: September 18, 2006
Branch: U.S. Army

Sergeant James R. Worster died September 18, 2006, of cardiac arrest in Baghdad, Iraq. The 24-year-old Army Medic was assigned to the 10th Combat Support Hospital, 43rd Area Support Group out of Fort Carson, Colorado, in support of Operation Iraqi Freedom. This was his second tour of duty in Iraq. In 2003, he served as a Field Medic. In accordance with his wishes, Worster was cremated.

James is survived by his wife, Brandy; his son, Trevor; his mother, Donna; two brothers, Jack and Josh; and his sister, Joy.

CHARLES D. ALLEN
Died: January 4, 2007
Branch: U.S. Army

Staff Sergeant Charles D. Allen was shot during combat operations in Baghdad, Iraq, on January 4, 2007. The 28-year-old Combat

Medic served with the 296th Brigade Support Battalion, 3rd Brigade Combat Team, 2nd Infantry Division out of Fort Lewis, Washington. He had volunteered to leave the safety of the base to assist an Infantry Battalion whose Medics needed a rest. On his first day with the Battalion, he was mortared while treating the wounded at the scene of a car bombing, made several runs to the field hospital under fire, and had a car bomb go off within 100 yards of his Stryker vehicle. He thanked the commander for the opportunity and asked if he could go back the next day. He is buried at Tahoma National Cemetery in Kent, Washington.

A memorial service in Wasilla, Alaska, drew about 200 people, including Governor Sarah Palin. Charles is survived by his wife Kerensa; son Orion; and parents David and Kathy.

JOHN E. ALLEN
Died: March 17, 2007
Branch: U.S. Army

Sergeant John E. Allen was killed March 17, 2007, when an improvised explosive device detonated near his vehicle during combat operations in Baghdad, Iraq. He was assigned to 2nd Battalion, 12th Cavalry Regiment, 4th Brigade Combat Team, 1st Cavalry Division, out of Fort Bliss, Texas, in support of Operation Iraqi Freedom. Allen was buried with full military honors in Arlington National Cemetery.

John was famous for his goofball sense of humor. A friend, Jim Johnson, described him this way: "All you had to do was ask him once, and he would be up there singing karaoke." His twin sister, Amanda, said, "He always created these special, funny moments. John had a way of making good things happen even though it was done in the strangest possible way."

John is survived by his wife, Aspen; his parents, Richard and Kellie; his twin sister, Amanda; and his brother, Adam.

BRIAN D. ALLGOOD
Died: January 20, 2007
Branch: U.S. Army

On January 20, 2007, Army Colonel Brian D. Allgood, the Command Surgeon, Milti-National Forces Iraq, turned over a new American built hospital to the people of Taji as part of an ongoing effort to rebuild the entire Iraqi health care system. On the return flight to Camp Victory in Baghdad, the Arkansas Army National Guard helicopter carrying Allgood and 11 other Soldiers was hit by a surface-to-air missle near the insurgent stronghold of Baqubah and crashed in Diyala Province northeast of Baghdad. All 12 Soldiers on board died. The most senior Army Medical Officer yet to die in Operation Iraqi Freedom, Allgood had been in this demanding post since July 2006. His future in the Army Medical Department seemed to be exceptionally bright, and he had been selected to assume command of the 30th Medical Brigade in Germany in the summer of 2007.

Memorial services were held at the Camp Liberty Chapel in Baghdad; Heidelberg, Germany; Fort Bragg, North Carolina; and Colorado Springs, Colorado, his hometown and the home of his parents. After memorial services in their hometowns, Brian and his Army colleagues who died in the crash were buried in a group interment at Arlington National Cemetery, on October 12, 2007.

He is survived by his wife Sallye; his son Wyatt; and his parents, Jerry and Cleo.

The son of a career Army Medical Service Corps Officer, Allgood was a 1982 graduate of the U.S. Military Academy. He attended the University of Oklahoma College of Medicine in Oklahoma City, following in the footsteps of his paternal grandfather and uncle. Upon receiving his M.D. in 1986, he entered the Army Medical Corps. He served a one-year internship in general surgery at Brooke Army Medical Center at Fort Sam Houston, Texas, before completing the Ranger and Combat Casualty Care courses. From 1987 to 1990, he was the Surgeon for the 3rd Battalion, 75th Ranger Regiment at Fort Benning, Georgia, and completed the Army Medical Department Officers Advanced, Army Flight Surgeon, and Jumpmaster courses. He jumped into Panama with his Battalion in December 1989 in Operation Just Cause and was awarded the Combat Medical Badge.

Allgood completed a four-year residency in orthopedic surgery at Brooke Army Medical Center and became the Division Orthopedic Surgeon for the 82nd Airborne Division at Fort Bragg, North Carolina, in 1994. In 1996, he achieved board certification in orthopedics and moved to Womack Army Medical Center at Fort Bragg, as Chief of the Orthopedic Clinic while also serving as the Orthopedic Consultant to the Joint Special Operations Command.

Brian's strong belief in the importance of religion and family made him a quiet, yet firm and confident leader.

To honor his legacy the U.S. Army Hospital located at Camp Humphreys, South Korea, is named the Brian D. Allgood Community Hospital.

RYAN J. BAUM
Died: May 18, 2007
Branch: U.S. Army

Sergeant Ryan J. Baum died May 18, 2007, in Karmah, Iraq, of wounds received from contact with enemy forces using small-arms fire. He was assigned to the 3rd Battalion, 509th Infantry Regiment, 4th Brigade Combat Team, 25th Infantry Division out of Fort Richardson, Alaska. Baum was scheduled to go home the day after he died. Hundreds attended the fallen Soldier's funeral held at Southeast Christian Church in Parker, Colorado.

In addition to his wife, Amber, and daughter Leia, Ryan is survived by his parents, Richard and Dana; his brother, Jason, and his sister, Mande.

CHRISTOPHER K. BOONE

Died: February 17, 2007
Branch: U.S. Army

Specialist Chris K. Boone died as the result of a non-combat related incident in Balad, Iraq, on February 17, 2007. The 34-year-old Medic served with the Georgia Army National Guard's H Company, 121st Infantry Long Range Surveillance Unit out of Fort Gillem, Georgia. His unit was protecting the border between Iraq and Syria. He was laid to rest at Houston National Cemetery in Houston, Texas.

MATTHEW C. BOWE

Died: February 19, 2007
Branch: U.S. Army

Private First Class Matthew C. Bowe, a Combat Medic, was killed on February 19, 2007, in Baghdad, Iraq, when the vehicle in which he was riding was struck by an IED. He was serving with the 1st Squadron, 89th Cavalry Regiment, 2nd Brigade Combat Team, 10th Mountain Division out of Fort Drum, New York. He was buried at Coraopolis Cemetery in Coraopolis, Pennsylvania. More than 250 people from his small hometown of Moon, Pennsylvania, attended his funeral.

Matt is survived by his parents, John and Lori; and siblings Melinda, Amanda, John, Megan and Tiffany.

JOSHUA M. BOYD

Died: March 14, 2007
Branch: U.S. Army

On March 14, 2007, Sergeant Joshua M. Boyd succumbed to wounds he received on March 5 when an improvised explosive device exploded near his vehicle in Samarra, Iraq. He was serving with C Company, 2nd Battalion, 505th Parachute Infantry Regiment, 3rd Brigade Combat Team, 82nd Airborne Division out of Fort Bragg,

North Carolina. Boyd died at Brook Army Medical Center, Fort Sam Houston, Texas. He was laid to rest in Elliott Hamil Garden of Memories in Abilene, Texas.

As a Combat Medic, Josh lived by a simple creed: to help those who could not help themselves. He was remembered by his friends as an active, intelligent man who loved to heal others.

Josh is survived by his parents, Robin and Tonya.

JONATHAN D. CADAVERO
Died: February 27, 2007
Branch: U.S. Army

Specialist Jonathan D. Cadavero was killed on February 27, 2007, when an improvised explosive device detonated near his vehicle in Baghdad, Iraq. He died while on an IED hunting mission in support of Operation Iraqi Freedom. The 24-year-old Combat Medic served with the 2nd Brigade Special Troops Battalion, 2nd Brigade Combat Team, 10th Mountain Division out of Fort Drum, New York. He was buried at the Orange County Veteran's Cemetery in Goshen, New Jersey.

Cadavero was a Medic with a platoon tasked with hunting IEDs and disposing of them before they could explode—one of the most vital and dangerous assignments in Iraq. In a six-month period, Cadavero's platoon found and disposed of 172 IEDs, 62 of which had the potential to explode.

Jon is survived by his wife, Michelle; his parents, Nadia and David; and his sister, Kristina.

MARK R. CANNON
Died: October 2, 2007
Branch: U.S. Navy

Petty Officer Third Class Mark R. Cannon was killed in action by a gunshot wound while on patrol in Kunar Province, Afghanistan, on October 2, 2007. He was assigned to the 3rd Battalion, 3rd Marine Regiment, 3rd Marine Division based out of Marine Corps Base

Hawaii. Cannon was buried at Saint Stephen's Episcopal Church in Lubbock, Texas.

Mark is survived by his father, Tom.

JOSEPH H. CANTRELL, IV
Died: April 4, 2007
Branch: U.S. Army

Corporal Joseph H. Cantrell, IV, paid the ultimate sacrifice when an improvised explosive device detonated near his vehicle in Taji, Iraq, on April 4, 2007. The 23-year-old served with the 2nd Battalion, 8th Cavalry Regiment, 1st Brigade Combat Team, 1st Cavalry Division out of Fort Hood, Texas. He was buried near his hometown of Westwood, Kentucky.

Joe is survived by his father, Joseph; his mother, Sondra; and his brother, Chase.

MATTHEW G. CONTE
Died: February 1, 2007
Branch: U.S. Navy

Hospital Corpsman Matthew G. Conte was killed February 1, 2007, when an IED exploded near his vehicle during combat operations in Anbar Province, Iraq. He was assigned to 2nd Battalion, 3rd Marine Regiment, 3rd Marine Division based in Kaneohe Bay, Hawaii. Funeral services were held on Saturday, February 24, 2007, at Grace Church of Rootstown, Ohio. Matt was cremated.

Inspired by patriotism, Conte joined the Navy in February 2004. He initially wanted to be a mason, but a long waiting list led him to become a Medic, a path more suited to his compassionate side. He had served in Afghanistan, and a friend recalled it had a strong effect on him. After the military, he planned to attend a radiology program and work at a hospital in his hometown.

Matt leaves behind his parents, Gale and Lureen; and his sister, Lora.

ERIC D. COTTRELL

Died: August 13, 2007
Branch: U.S. Army

Staff Sergeant Eric D. Cottrell was killed on August 13, 2007, when an improvised explosive device struck his vehicle in Qayyarah, Iraq. The 39-year-old served with the 5th Battalion, 82nd Field Artillery Regiment, 4th Brigade Combat Team, 1st Cavalry Division out of Fort Bliss, Texas. Cottrell was buried with full military honors at Fort Mitchell National Cemetery in Fort Mitchell, Alabama.

In remarks read on the floor of the U.S. House of Representatives, California Representative Ken Calvert marveled at Cottrell's devotion to his fellow Soldiers. He had clearly earned their respect because they called him "Doc." Cotrell was right there on the front lines, ready to help his brothers in arms who had been hurt.

Eric is survived by his wife, Sherri; two daughters, Megan and Brandy; two sons, James and Eric; his parents, Alan and Mannie; and two brothers, Norris and Christopher.

CARLETTA S. DAVIS

Died: November 5, 2007
Branch: U.S. Army

Staff Sergeant Carletta S. Davis was killed on November 5, 2007, in Tal Al-Dahab, Iraq, when an improvised explosive device detonated near her Humvee during combat operations. The 34-year-old medic served with the 10th Brigade Support Battalion, 1st Brigade Combat Team, 10th Mountain Division out of Fort Drum, New York. She was buried at a small family service at the Northern Lights Memorial Cemetery in Fairbanks, Alaska. She had received full military honors at several previous memorial services.

Davis was an accomplished Medic, and always looked out for those under her protection. She was selected as lead Medic in the Brigade Commander's personal security detachment, an elite position that often took her away from her fortified base near Kirkuk. She received two awards for heroism: the first for rescuing two Soldiers who had fallen down a cliff near Fort Lewis, Washington, and a second for rescuing a wounded Iraqi police officer.

Carletta is survived by her husband, Thomas; three sons, Treyton, Theodore, and Tyrique; and mother, Lavada.

SCOTT E. DUFFMAN
Died: February 17, 2007
Branch: U.S. Air Force

Air Force Technical Sergeant Scott E. Duffman was killed on February 17, 2007, in a helicopter crash in eastern Afghanistan during Operation Enduring Freedom. The Chinook helicopter carrying Duffman and 21 other military personnel was en route from Kandahar to Bagram when it crashed in the Zabula Province of Afghanistan, killing 8 and injuring 14. Technical Sergeant Duffman was buried with full military honors at Arlington National Cemetery. Mourners gathered to pay their respects to the fallen hero.

Duffman was a decorated Airman. Though his military career was cut short, he earned the Bronze Star with Valor, the Defense Meritorious Service Medal, the Air Medal, and numerous awards of the Air Force Commendation Medals and Air Force Achievement Medals.

Scott leaves behind his wife, Mary; his newborn daughter, Sophia; and his mother, Rose.

NICHOLAS D. EISCHEN
Died: December 25, 2007
Branch: U.S. Air Force

Senior Airman Nicholas D. Eischen of the U.S. Air Force died in his sleep on December 25, 2007, at Bagram Air Base in Afghanistan. The 24-year-old Medic was assigned to the 60th Medical Operations Squadron based at Travis Air Force Base, California, and was bravely serving his country in support of Operation Enduring Freedom. About 500 family, friends, and members of the community gathered on January 4, 2008, at New Hope Community Church in Clovis, California, to say their final farewells.

Nick leaves behind his wife, Leah; a young son, Braeden; parents, Drew and Suzi; and his sister, Jaime.

LUCAS W. A. EMCH
Died: March 2, 2007
Branch: U.S. Navy

Navy Hospital Corpsman Lucas W. A. Emch was killed on March 2, 2007, in Al Anbar Province, Iraq. His death resulted from injuries sustained from the detonation of a makeshift bomb while he was conducting combat operations in support of Operation Iraqi Freedom. He was assigned as a Hospital Corpsman to the 1st Marine Logistics Group, I Marine Expeditionary Force based at Camp Pendleton, California. Funeral services for the 21-year-old Sailor were held on March 12, 2007, at the Donovan Funeral Home in Tallmadge, Ohio. He was buried with full military honors at the Ohio Western Reserve National Cemetery in Rittman, Ohio.

Surviving Luke are his parents, Wesley and Julie; his sister, Samantha; and his grandparents, Albert and Jean.

GLADE L. FELIX
Died: June 11, 2007
Branch: U.S. Air Force

Lieutenant Colonel Glade L. Felix of the United States Air Force Reserve died of heart complications on June 11, 2007, at Al Udeid Air Base in Qatar. The 52-year-old officer was a reservist with the 622nd Aeromedical Staging Squadron at Robins Air Force Base in Georgia; he was in Qatar serving with the 379th Expeditionary Medical Group in support of Operation Iraqi Freedom. He was buried in Evergreen Cemetery in Utah on June 21, 2007.

He leaves behind his wife, Cathie; and their six children, Chris, Leo, Chelsea, Jim, Katie, and Sean.

MICHAEL S. FIELDER

Died: August 19, 2007
Branch: U.S. Army

Captain Michael S. Fielder gave his life in service to his country on August 19, 2007, in Baghdad, Iraq. In support of Operation Iraqi Freedom, he proudly served with the 248th Medical Detachment, 44th Medical Command, 18th Airborne Corps out of Fort Bragg, North Carolina. He died in a non-combat related incident. A celebration of his life was held at Hudson Memorial Church in Raleigh, North Carolina.

Mike is survived by his wife, Mary; and his mother, Janet.

GABRIEL J. FIGUEROA

Died: April 3, 2007
Branch: U.S. Army

Private First Class Gabriel Figueroa sacrificed his life for his country when he was shot by a sniper during combat operations in Baghdad, Iraq, on April 3, 2007. He proudly served with the 1st Battalion, 8th Cavalry Regiment, 2nd Brigade Combat Team, 1st Cavalry Division out of Fort Hood, Texas. When he was shot, this cheerful and caring Soldier was handing out candy and toys to Iraqi children. As a testament to the love and impact Figueroa had on his community, more than 700 people gathered for his service. Figueroa's family laid their son to rest with full military honors at Rose Hills Memorial Park in Whittier, California.

Gabriel was a thoughtful and funny young man, enjoying fishing and reading in his spare time. While in high school, he also volunteered at the local hospital, visiting the sick and assisting nurses with their duties.

Gabriel particularly enjoyed it when his fellow Soldiers called him "Doc," and they depended upon him for their well-being. He made many friends while in the Army and they all have the same sentiment for their battle buddy, their Doc, and their friend. He will forever remain in their hearts as a true American hero.

Gabriel is survived by his parents, Javier and Elsa; two brothers, Xavier and Sebastian; and two sisters, Danica and Tanya.

JOSEPH GILMORE
Died: May 19, 2007
Branch: U.S. Army

Specialist Joseph Gilmore died from wounds received when an improvised explosive device detonated near his vehicle in Baghdad, Iraq, on May 19, 2007. The 26-year-old Medic served with the 1st Battalion, 5th Cavalry Regiment, 2nd Brigade Combat Team, 1st Cavalry Division out of Fort Hood, Texas. Gilmore chose to be cremated and his ashes were spread in multiple locations in Alaska.

Joseph is survived by his wife, Eve; and two children.

DANIEL E. GOMEZ
Died: July 18, 2007
Branch: U.S. Army

Specialist Daniel E. Gomez gave his life in service to his country on July 18, 2007, when his vehicle was attacked in Adhamiyah, Iraq. The enemy employed a makeshift bomb and small-arms fire against Gomez's unit. He served with the 1st Battalion, 26th Infantry Regiment, 2nd Brigade Combat Team, 1st Infantry Division out of Schweinfurt, Germany. At Gomez's request, his family laid their eldest son to rest in San Antonio, Texas, close to where he had trained to be a Medic. He was buried with full military honors in the Fort Sam Houston National Cemetery.

His parents remember their son as a "big-hearted person" who wanted to care for everyone, both American and Iraqi. They are grateful for the outpouring of support they received from people around the world whose lives Daniel had touched. In an email to his sister about a week before he died, Daniel stressed his role as a Soldier to protect all of the United States, and to see the mission through to the end:

If I ever go to war, Mom, please don't be afraid. There are some things I must do to keep the promise that I made. I'm sure there will be some heartache, and I know that you'll cry tears. But your son is a Soldier now, Mom, there is nothing you should fear. If I ever go to war, Dad, I know that you'll be strong. But you won't have to worry, cause you taught me right from wrong. You kept me firmly on the ground, yet still taught me how to fly. Your son is a Soldier now, Dad, I love you, hooah, even if I die. If I ever go to war, Bro, there are some things I want to say. You've always had my back, and I know it's my time to repay. You'll always be my daybreak, through all of life's dark clouds, your brother is a Soldier now, Bro, I promise I'll make you proud. If I ever go to war Sis, don't you worry about me, I always looked out for you, but I can't do that anymore, Cause I am a big bro to all in America. I love you so much and you know that your brother is a Soldier now, Sis, so wipe your eyes, I'll be fine even if I die. If I ever go to war my friends, we'll never be apart, though we may not meet again, I'll hold you in my heart. Remember all the times we had, don't let your memories cease, your friend is a Soldier now dear friend, and I'll die to bring you peace. And when I go to Heaven, and see that pearly gate, I'll gladly decline entrance, then stand my post and wait. I'm sorry, Sir, I can't come in, I'm sort of in a bind, you see I'm still a Soldier, Sir, so I can't leave them behind.
- *Written by Daniel E. Gomez to his family and friends.*

Daniel is survived by his parents, Juan and Juanita; his sister Marian; and his brother Louie.

JOSHUA S. HARMON
Died: August 22, 2007
Branch: U.S. Army

Corporal Joshua S. Harmon died on August 22, 2007, when his UH-60 Black Hawk helicopter crashed at Multaka near Kirkuk,

Iraq. At the time of his death, Harmon was a Combat Medic assigned to the 2nd Battalion, 35th Infantry Regiment, 3rd Infantry Brigade Combat Team, 25th Infantry Division based out of Schofield Barracks, Hawaii. This was his first tour of duty in Iraq. Harmon was laid to rest in Mentor Municipal Cemetery in his hometown of Mentor, Ohio.

Josh is survived by his wife, Kristin; parents, Donna and Richard; and his brother, Jason.

ROSELLE M. HOFFMASTER
Died: September 20, 2007
Branch: U.S. Army

Captain Roselle M. Hoffmaster was killed on September 20, 2007, in Kirkuk, Iraq, supporting Operation Iraqi Freedom. She died of injuries sustained in a non-combat related incident. As a Brigade Surgeon, Hoffmaster was assigned to HQ Company, 1st Brigade Combat Team, 10th Mountain Division out of Fort Drum, New York. Her family held memorial services for her on September 29, 2007, in West Chester, Pennsylvania.

Roselle is survived by her husband, Gordon, and her parents.

DARREN P. HUBBELL
Died: June 20, 2007
Branch: U.S. Army

Staff Sergeant Darren P. Hubbell gave his life in service to his country on June 20, 2007, in Baghdad, Iraq, when a roadside bomb exploded near his vehicle. He served with the 1st Battalion, 64th Armor Regiment, 2nd Brigade Combat Team, 3rd Infantry Division out of Fort Stewart, Georgia. Hubbell was buried in Christian Life Fellowship Church Cemetery in his hometown of Metter, Georgia. Residents of the small town lined the streets as the funeral procession brought his body back home from Savannah, Georgia.

A 14-year veteran, this Senior Line Medic had also served tours in Panama and Afghanistan. At the time of his death, he was on his third tour in Iraq. In fact, Hubbell was involved with the first wave of U.S. Troops into Iraq. His Brigade was one of the first to enter and take over Baghdad.

Darren is survived by his wife, Dana; a son, Darren, Jr.; a daughter, Marina; and his father, Gary.

RACHAEL L. HUGO
Died: October 5, 2007
Branch: U.S. Army

Corporal Rachael L. Hugo was killed on October 5, 2007, when a roadside bomb hit her convoy outside Baiji, Iraq, just north of Baghdad, while they were on a supply run. Although Hugo was evacuated, she died at the hospital after receiving last rites. Hugo was a Combat Medic assigned to the Army Reserve's 303rd Military Police Company, 97th Military Police Battalion, 89th Military Police Brigade based in Jackson, Michigan. She was buried at Roselawn Memorial Park in Menona, Wisconsin, on October 18, 2007, with full military honors.

Hugo was a dedicated Medic. From Iraq, she wrote her family, "This is what I choose to do, and being a Medic is what I live to do." Her father remembered that she "was always very adamant about volunteering and going out on missions with her guys. She told us countless times that she needed to be there with them. If somebody got hurt and they didn't have a Medic, she was beside herself." Her mother said, "She felt that was her niche in life, helping people."

Rachael is survived by her parents, Kermit and Ruth; and her younger brother, Scott.

MICHAEL R. HULLENDER
Died: April 28, 2007
Branch: U.S. Army

Staff Sergeant Michael R. Hullender died April 28, 2007, when he stepped on a land mine while assisting a wounded Soldier. The 29-year-old served as a Ranger and Medic in the 1st Battalion, 501st

Airborne Infantry Regiment, 4th Brigade Combat Team, 25th Infantry Division out of Fort Richardson, Alaska. He was buried with full military honors in Broadlawn Memorial Gardens in Buford, Georgia.

The August after he died, the University of West Georgia awarded Michael a posthumous Bachelor of Business Administration degree. When he enlisted in the Army, he had attended the college for about two years, and he promised his parents that he would finish his degree. The college awarded the degree in recognition of that promise.

Mike is survived by his father, Ren; his mother, Cindy; his two older sisters, Lisa and Amy; and his fiancée, Kylee.

SHIN W. KIM
Died: June 28, 2007
Branch: U.S. Army

Sergeant Shin W. Kim was killed on June 28, 2007, when insurgents using makeshift bombs in Baghdad, Iraq, attacked his unit. Only 23 years old, the young medic served with the 2nd Battalion, 12th Infantry Regiment, 2nd Brigade Combat Team, 2nd Infantry Division out of Fort Carson, Colorado. Kim's brother, Josh, said he did not die immediately from the attack. A doctor in Iraq held a telephone to Kim's ear as his family bid their hero goodbye. At his gravesite, hundreds of mourners released white balloons into the sky in his honor. He was buried with full military honors at Rose Hills Memorial Park in Whittier, California.

Shin is survived by his parents, Yoo Buk and Kum Ok; brother, Josh; sister, Shinae; and girlfriend, Tammy.

GARRETT C. KNOLL
Died: April 23, 2007
Branch: U.S. Army

Private First Class Garrett C. Knoll died on April 23, 2007, of wounds he suffered when a suicide car bomber detonated an IED next to his patrol base in As Sadah, Iraq. Eight other Soldiers were killed and 20 more were wounded in the deadliest single incident for the 82nd Airborne since the Vietnam War. The 23-year-old Combat Medic served with the 5th Squadron, 73rd Cavalry Regiment, 3rd Brigade Combat Team, 82nd Airborne Division out of Fort Bragg, North Carolina. Hundreds of family, friends, and members of the community of Bad Axe, Michigan, gathered on May 4, 2007, at the Bad Axe High School to honor their fallen hero. He was buried in the Verona Cemetery in Verona, Michigan.

Garrett is survived by his grandparents, Robert and Ruth, who raised him.

NICHOLAS J. LIGHTNER
Died: March 21, 2007
Branch: U.S. Army

Sergeant Nicholas J. Lightner was wounded on March 15, 2007, when a makeshift bomb detonated near his unit on a combat patrol in Baghdad, Iraq. He died of his wounds on March 21, 2007, at Walter Reed Army Medical Center in Washington, DC. The 29-year-old served with the 1st Squadron, 8th Cavalry Regiment, 2nd Brigade Combat Team, 1st Cavalry Division out of Fort Hood, Texas. On his deathbed, the dedicated Medic worried about the Soldiers he was unable to save. Even after he was wounded, Sergeant Lightner was able to save one other Soldier long enough for him to get to a hospital; tragically that Soldier died three days later. Hundreds of mourners attended Lightner's funeral service, which was held at Bateman Funeral Home in Newport, Oregon, on March 30, 2007.

Nick is survived by his father, Bill; brothers, Joshua and Nathan; and fiancée, Ginger.

PATRICK MAGNANI
Died: September 4, 2007
Branch: U.S. Air Force

Air Force Master Sergeant Patrick D. Magnani, a Biomedical Technician, died on September 4, 2007, in a non-combat related incident near Bagram Air Base, Afghanistan. The highly respected

38-year-old was assigned to the 31st Medical Support Squadron from Aviano Air Base, Italy. Friends and family gathered on September 12, 2007, in Pleasant Hill, California, to celebrate his life. He was buried in the Sacramento Valley Veteran's National Cemetery.

Patrick is survived by his parents, Thomas and Jeanne; brothers, Michael and Christopher; and sister, Katie.

CONOR G. MASTERSON
Died: April 8, 2007
Branch: U.S. Army

Corporal Conor G. Masterson died April 8, 2007, when an IED detonated near the patrol vehicle in which he was riding. The 21-year-old was serving with B Company, 1st Battalion, 4th Infantry Regiment out of Hohenfels, Germany, supporting Operation Enduring Freedom. He was laid to rest in Fort Snelling National Cemetery in Minneapolis, Minnesota.

The year after her son's death, Sandy Masterson began raising money to support the troops and their families with two other women who were similarly affected by the war in Iraq. A portion of the proceeds from their "Scoops for Troops" event was donated to Tribute to the Troops.

Conor is survived by his wife, Lorena; parents, Sandy and Mark; and siblings, Evan, Adam, Abbie, Christopher, Matthew, and Justin.

MARQUIS J. MCCANTS
Died: May 18, 2007
Branch: U.S. Army

Specialist Marquis J. McCants was killed in Baghdad, Iraq, on May 18, 2007, when his unit was attacked with an improvised explosive device and small-arms fire. He was serving with the 1st Battalion, 325th Airborne Infantry Regiment, 2nd Brigade Combat Team, 82nd Airborne Division out of Fort Bragg, North Carolina. He was buried with full military honors at Fort Sam Houston National Cemetery, San Antonio, Texas, on Memorial Day weekend.

Marquis is survived by his wife, Andrea; children, Azaria and Micah; parents, Savage and Belinda; brothers, Savage III, and Isaiah; and sisters, Patrice, Lisa, and Brandi.

GRAHAM M. MCMAHON
Died: September 19, 2007
Branch: U.S. Army

Corporal Graham M. McMahon died September 19, 2007, in Baghdad, Iraq, from a non-combat related illness. The 22-year-old Medic served with the 4th Battalion, 9th Infantry Regiment, 4th Stryker Brigade Combat Team, 2nd Infantry Division out of Fort Lewis, Washington. After returning from patrol with his unit, McMahon suddenly became ill and died en route to the hospital. A public memorial service was held in the auditorium at the Benton County Fairgrounds in Corvallis, Oregon.

Graham leaves behind his wife, Angelique; his father, Bill; and his brother, Dylan.

PHILLIP D. MCNEILL
Died: January 20, 2007
Branch: U.S. Army

Sergeant Phillip D. McNeill died when an improvised explosive device detonated near his Humvee in Karmah, Iraq, on January 20, 2007. Three other Soldiers died in the same incident. The 22-year-old Combat Medic was serving with the 3rd Battalion, 509th Parachute Infantry Regiment, 4th Brigade Combat Team, 25th Infantry Division out of Fort Richardson, Alaska. He was laid to rest in Owingsville Cemetery in Owingsville, Kentucky.

Phillip is survived by his parents, David and Angela; his brother, Chris; and his fiancée Cassandra.

HUGO V. MENDOZA
Died: October 25, 2007
Branch: U.S. Army

Specialist Hugo V. Mendoza died on October 25, 2007, from wounds received during an ambush in the Korengal Valley, Afghanistan. The 29-year-old Combat Medic died under a hail of rocket propelled grenades, machine gun fire, and small-arms as he tried to save wounded Soldiers being dragged away by Taliban forces. Specialist Mendoza threw grenades at the enemy, preventing them from taking the Soldier, who was also killed in the attack. He was laid to rest with full military honors at Fort Bliss National Cemetery in El Paso, Texas.

Mendoza's fellow Soldiers knew that the infantryman would stand beside them until the call for a Medic was heard. Then he became "Doc," the man who would run out into the fray to care for a wounded comrade with no concern for his own safety.

Hugo is survived by his parents, Jesus and Sara; and his brother, Jesus, Jr.

CHARLES L. MILAM
Died: September 25, 2007
Branch: U.S. Navy

Petty Officer Second Class Charles L. Milam, a Navy Hospital Corpsman, died September 25, 2007, while serving in support of Operation Enduring Freedom. The 26-year-old Sailor was killed in an ambush rocket attack while patrolling an opium poppy growing area with coalition forces in Helmand Province, Afghanistan. Milam was assigned to the 2nd Marine Special Operations Battalion at Camp Lejeune, North Carolina. He was laid to rest with full military honors at Fort Logan National Cemetery in Denver, Colorado.

It is clear that Luke was devoted to his calling. "He had served three tours in Iraq, and would have gone back however many times it took to get the job done," his brother Keith said. "He felt it was his duty to do whatever he could to help people in the military. He was a hero in every sense of the term." Luke's sister said, "He loved what he did. He loved his guys and would have done anything for them."

Luke is survived by his parents, Michael and Rita; his brothers, Keith and Andrew; and his sister, Jaime.

GILBERT MINJARES, JR.
Died: February 7, 2007
Branch: U.S. Navy

Petty Officer First Class "Beto" Minjares, Jr., a Navy Hospital Corpsman, died on February 7, 2007, when his helicopter was shot down by enemy fire while his unit was conducting operations in Anbar Province, Iraq. Assigned to the Marine Aircraft Group 14, 2nd Marine Aircraft Wing in Cherry Point, North Carolina, the 31-year-old Sailor had been in Iraq only several days at the time of his death. Funeral services were held on February 20, 2007, at Saint Raphael's Catholic Church in El Paso, Texas.

On March 19, 2008, Beto's family got together to celebrate what would have been his 33rd birthday. His wife Jeannie helped their children, Gilbert and Miranda make a birthday cake and sing "Happy Birthday." Jeannie said she tells their children every day about their father.

Beto leaves behind his wife, Jeannie; a son, Gilbert, III; his daughter Miranda, just a newborn when her father died; his parents, Gilbert and Rosa; sisters, Zonia, Aurora, and Laura; and his brother Jose.

DAN H. NGUYEN
Died: May 8, 2007
Branch: U.S. Army

Specialist Dan H. Nguyen sacrificed his life for his country when he was fatally wounded during an attack by enemy small-arms fire in Tahrir, Iraq, on May 8, 2007. He died while trying to rescue a fellow Soldier during the gun battle. The 24-year-old Medic served with the 1st Battalion, 12th Cavalry Regiment, 3rd Brigade Combat Team, 1st Cavalry Division out of Fort Hood, Texas. Mourners gathered to remember him on May 26, 2007, at the Christ Incarnate Word Catholic Church in Houston, Texas. Specialist Nguyen was laid to rest with full military honors in the Houston National Cemetery.

Dan is survived by his parents, Sony and Huong; his fiancée, Hau; and his brothers, Phi, Vu, and Van.

DANIEL S. NOBLE
Died: July 24, 2007
Branch: U.S. Navy

Hospital Corpsman Daniel S. Noble was killed July 24, 2007, by an improvised explosive device while conducting security operations in the Diyala Province of Iraq, in support of Operation Iraqi Freedom. He was assigned to K Battery, 3rd Battalion, 12th Marine Regiment, 1st Marine Division. His family and friends paid their respects to him on August 1, 2007, at the Rose Hills Memorial Park in Whittier, California, where he was buried with full military honors.

Daniel is survived by his parents, Barry and Julie; his brother, Andrew; and his sister, Katlin.

MARIA I. ORTIZ
Died: July 10, 2007
Branch: U.S. Army

Army Nurse Corps Captain Maria I. Ortiz was returning to her barracks after physical training on July 10, 2007, when she was killed by shrapnel from a mortar attack. The 40-year-old was the first female Army Nurse killed in combat since the Vietnam War. At the time of her death, she was assigned to the 28th Combat Support Hospital located in the Green Zone in Baghdad, Iraq.

Colleagues held a memorial service for her there and shared stories of how she touched their lives. Another ceremony took place on July 18, 2007, at Aberdeen Proving Grounds, Maryland, where Maria formerly served. A pair of combat boots, a helmet, and Ortiz's dog tags were arranged on the Post Chapel's altar. Many came forward to salute the display. Hundreds of mourners bid farewell to their loving Army Nurse at Arlington National Cemetery on August 9, 2007, where a horse-drawn caisson carried Ortiz to her final resting place. An honor guard then rendered a 21-gun salute in a tribute to her.

Maria is survived by her parents, Jorge and Iris; her four sisters, including her twin, Maria; and her fiancée, Juan.

TIMOTHY P. PADGETT
Died: May 8, 2007
Branch: U.S. Army

Special Forces Sergeant Timothy P. Padgett died for his country on May 8, 2007, while serving in Operation Enduring Freedom, when Taliban fighters fired guns, grenades, and mortars at his Special Forces team while they were conducting a combat patrol in Tarin Kwot, Afghanistan. Padgett died from wounds he received during the firefight. The 28-year-old Green Beret was assigned to 1st Battalion, 7th Special Forces Group out of Fort Bragg, North Carolina. Funeral services for the fallen hero were held on May 16, 2007, at the First United Methodist Church in DeFuniak Springs, Florida, after which he was laid to rest with full military honors.

Tim is survived by his daughter, Summer; his mother, Glenda; his father, Tommy; his sister, Serena; his brother, Rex; and his fiancée, Stacey.

JAVIER G. PAREDES
Died: September 5, 2007
Branch: U.S. Army

Corporal Javier G. Paredes was killed on September 5, 2007, by a rocket propelled grenade in Baghdad, Iraq. The 24-year-old Medic served with the 2nd Battalion, 69th Armor Regiment, 3rd Brigade Combat Team, 3rd Infantry Division out of Fort Benning, Georgia. Family and friends paid their last respects on September 14, 2007, at the St. Patrick Catholic Church in San Antonio, Texas. Paredes was laid to rest with full military honors at the Fort Sam Houston National Cemetery.

Paredes found a home in the Army in 2004 and became a dedicated Soldier after having overcome an abusive and neglectful childhood, passing through a series of foster homes, and often separated from his four brothers.

Javier is survived by his Aunt Maria, and his four brothers.

JUAN S. RESTREPO
Died: July 22, 2007
Branch: U.S. Army

Private First Class Juan S. Restrepo made the ultimate sacrifice for his adopted country on July 22, 2007, in Korengal Valley, Afghanistan. The 20-year-old Airborne Combat Medic died of injuries he received when his dismounted patrol came under small-arms fire. Restrepo served with the 2nd Battalion, 503rd Infantry Regiment, 173rd Airborne Brigade Combat Team out of Vicenza, Italy. Funeral services were held in his native country of Colombia.

Juan leaves behind many family and friends to cherish his memory.

JONATHAN RIVADENEIRA
Died: September 14, 2007
Branch: U.S. Army

Specialist Jonathan Rivadeneira was killed on September 14, 2007, when an improvised explosive device detonated near his vehicle while conducting combat operations in Baghdad, Iraq. The 22-year-old Combat Medic was assigned to the 6th Squadron, 9th Cavalry Regiment, 3rd Brigade Combat Team, 1st Cavalry Division out of Fort Hood, Texas. Rivadeneira served his unit with dedication and valor, volunteering to accompany his unit on the front lines rather than remaining in the safety of the aid station. About 200 friends and family gathered to say their final farewells to their husband, son, friend, and Soldier on September 25, 2007, at St. Joan of Arc Church in Jackson Heights, New York. He was laid to rest in St. Michael's Cemetery in Astoria, New York.

Jonathan is survived by his wife, Heather; and his mother, Martha.

LESTER G. ROQUE

Died: November 10, 2007
Branch: U.S. Army

Specialist Lester G. Roque died on November 10, 2007, as a result of wounds sustained in support of Operation Enduring Freedom. Direct enemy fire hit Roque's patrol in Aranus, Afghanistan, on November 9, 2007. Several Soldiers lost their lives in the same incident. The 23-year-old Medic served with the 2nd Battalion, 503rd Airborne Infantry Regiment, 173rd Airborne Brigade Combat Team based in Vincenza, Italy. Lester's family held a viewing of his casket on the 22nd and 23rd of November, 2007. Lester was laid to rest with full military honors in Forest Lawn Memorial Park in Cypress.

Lester is survived by his parents, Antonio and Clarissa; his brother Leo; and his fiancée, Leikathryn.

MANUEL A. RUIZ

Died: February 7, 2007
Branch: U.S. Navy

Petty Officer Third Class Manuel A. Ruiz died on February 7, 2007, in Al Anbar Province, Iraq, from injuries sustained in a helicopter accident. He was a passenger in the CH-46 Sea Knight helicopter that experienced difficulties about 20 miles northwest of Baghdad. Seven military personnel died in the crash. The failure of the aircraft was attributed to either mechanical malfunction or hostile fire. Ruiz was assigned to the 2nd Medical Battalion, 2nd Marine Logistics Group out of Camp Lejeune, North Carolina. On February 21, 2007, a viewing was held at the Frampton Funeral Home in Federalsburg, Maryland. On February 22, the 21-year-old was laid to rest with full military honors at Arlington National Cemetery.

Manuel is survived by his parents, Manuel and Lisa; and his brothers, Joshua and Jacob.

RYAN D. RUSSELL
Died: March 5, 2007
Branch: U.S. Army

Specialist Ryan D. Russell sacrificed his life for his country on March 5, 2007, while caring for wounded fellow Soldiers in Baqubah, Iraq. The 20-year-old Medic was serving with the 1st Squadron, 12th Cavalry Regiment, 3rd Brigade Combat Team, 1st Cavalry Division based out of Fort Hood, Texas. He was providing lifesaving assistance to his injured comrades after an improvised explosive device hit one of his unit's Humvees. Russell was struck and killed when a second bomb detonated. A memorial ceremony was held in Russell's honor at the Nashville Praise and Worship Center, Nashville, North Carolina, and he was buried in Ayden Cemetery, Ayden, North Carolina.

Ryan is survived by his mother and his brother Robert. As a tribute to Ryan, his family established a memorial fund and asked his family and friends to donate to Give2TheTroops in Greenville, North Carolina, in his name.

BENJAMIN L. SEBBAN
Died: March 17, 2007
Branch: U.S. Army

Sergeant First Class Ben L. Sebban died on March 17, 2007, while serving in Baqubah, Iraq. In his Memorial Day 2007 radio address, President George W. Bush described Sebban's heroism. He said, "In Iraq's Diyala Province, Ben saw a truck filled with explosives racing toward his team of paratroopers. He ran into the open to warn them, exposing himself to the blast. Ben received severe wounds, but this good medic never bothered to check his own injuries. Instead, he devoted his final moments on this earth to treating others." A memorial service in his honor took place on March 28, 2007, at Christ

Church in South Amboy, New Jersey. He was buried the following day at Arlington National Cemetery.

Ben is survived by his mother, Barbara; and his brothers, Daniel and David.

ASHLEY SIETSEMA
Died: November 12, 2007
Branch: U.S. Army

Specialist Ashley Sietsema died while she was serving her country in support of Operation Iraqi Freedom on November 12, 2007, in Kuwait City, Kuwait. Specialist Sietsema, an Army Medic and ambulance driver, was conducting a routine medical transfer of a patient from Camp Buehring to Camp Arifjan when she was involved in a single vehicle accident. The 20-year-old Combat Medic was part of the Illinois National Guard out of North Riverside, Illinois. Mourners gathered on November 18, 2007, to say their farewells at the Ronan-Moore Funeral Home in DeKalb, Illinois. She was laid to rest with full military honors in Fairview Park Cemetery.

Ashley is survived by her husband, Max; her mother, Olivia; and her brother, Kyle.

LANCE C. SPRINGER, II
Died: March 23, 2007
Branch: U.S. Army

Sergeant Lance Springer, II, died on March 23, 2007, from wounds he received when an improvised explosive device detonated near his unit. At the time he was on a combat patrol in Baghdad, Iraq. The 23-year-old was assigned to the 1st Squadron, 40th Cavalry Regiment, 4th Airborne Brigade Combat Team, 25th Infantry Division out of Fort Richardson, Alaska. Friends and family said their final goodbyes at Lakeside Church of God in Fort Worth, Texas. He was buried with full military honors at the Dallas-Fort Worth National Cemetery.

His family says he had a childhood dream of becoming a Soldier and was extremely proud of his military service. His father recalled that he always wanted to be a Soldier. He always loved the Army, his whole life. Lance added that his son supported his country in its efforts to help the Iraqi people.

Lance is survived by his parents, Lance and Evanna; his brother, Christopher; and his sister, Michelle.

DAVID A. STEPHENS
Died: April 12, 2007
Branch: U.S. Army

Sergeant David Alex Stephens gave his life in service to his country on April 12, 2007, when his vehicle was struck by an improvised explosive device during combat operations in Miri, Afghanistan. The 28-year-old Medic served with the 2nd Battalion, 508th Parachute Infantry Regiment, 4th Brigade Combat Team with the 82nd Airborne Division out of Fort Bragg, North Carolina. The Tennessee native was laid to rest in Pennington Cemetery in Franklin County, Tennessee.

As the funeral procession headed to Pennington Cemetery, Alex's family saw their wonderful community honor him respectfully as the hero he was. People lined the streets; 1,000 flags flew along the roadside; men, women, and children covered their hearts and waved flags. This display helped Alex's family realize the true meaning of community: "In our time of tragedy, we felt comfort and blessed to witness all this."

Alex leaves behind his wife, Megan, and his three-month-old daughter, Sienna; and his father, Charles.

JOHN S. STEPHENS
Died: March 15, 2007
Branch: U.S. Army

Sergeant First Class John S. Stephens was killed when his patrol came under enemy attack in Tikrit, Iraq, on March 15, 2007. He was serving with the 1st Battalion, 16th Infantry Regiment, 1st Brigade,

1st Infantry Division out of Fort Riley, Kansas. Stephens was driving a command vehicle when it was hit by an IED. His funeral service took place in his hometown of La Grande, Oregon, on March 26, 2007. He was escorted by Patriot Guard Riders to his final resting place in Grandview Cemetery.

John is survived by his wife, Beate; his children, Darren, Brian, and Cheryl; his parents, Gene and Eva; and his sister, Michelle.

DAVID T. TOOMALATAI

Died: January 27, 2007
Branch: U.S. Army

Private First Class David T. Toomalatai gave his life for his country on January 27, 2007, when the ambulance he was riding in rolled over a land mine in Taji, Iraq, while on a mission to pick up injured Soldiers. The 19-year-old Combat Medic was serving with the 2nd Battalion, 8th Cavalry Regiment, 1st Brigade Combat Team, 1st Cavalry Division out of Fort Hood, Texas, in support of Operation Iraqi Freedom. He had been in Iraq for only a few months at the time of his death. Family and friends laid him to rest in Green Hills Memorial Park in Rancho Palos Verdes, California.

Following in the footsteps of his retired Army father, and motivated by education benefits the Army has to offer, Toomalatai saw the Army as a way to provide for his family. He enlisted shortly after high school and completed boot camp at Fort Benning, Georgia, before training as a Medic at Fort Sam Houston, Texas.

David is survived by his son, Damien; his parents, Vai and Sally; his brothers and sisters, Savali, Doreen, Elizabeth, Mara, James, and Michael.

MICHAEL J. TULLY

Died: August 23, 2007
Branch: U.S. Army

Sergeant First Class Michael J. Tully was killed on August 23, 2007, at Al Aziziyah, southeast of Baghdad, Iraq, when a makeshift bomb exploded near his vehicle. Tully was assigned to C Company, 2nd Battalion, 1st Special Forces Group out of Fort Lewis, Washington. His body was escorted home by his brother John, also serving in Iraq. He was buried with full military honors at Beechwoods Cemetery in Falls Creek, Pennsylvania.

Michael is remembered by friends and family for his caring and compassionate nature. His father treasures a photograph of his son comforting a young Iraqi girl suffering from burns: "You could see his hand reaching for her to say, 'Honey, don't be afraid.'" Jack Tully also remembers that during Michael's training in U.S. hospitals, he delivered a baby one night. "That night represents one of the happiest moments of Michael's life," his father said.

Michael is survived by his wife, Heather; his son, Slade; his father, Jack; his mother, Dolores; his brother, John; and his sister, Heather.

DUSTIN S. WAKEMAN
Died: August 4, 2007
Branch: U.S. Army

Sergeant Dustin S. Wakeman died on August 4, 2007, in Hawr Rajab, Iraq, when an improvised explosive device struck the vehicle he was riding in during combat operations. He was serving with the 1st Squadron, 40th Cavalry Regiment, 4th Brigade Combat Team, 25th Infantry Division out of Fort Richardson, Alaska. He was laid to rest with full military honors on August 13, 2007, in the Laurel Land Memorial Park in Fort Worth, Texas.

Wakeman joined the Army in 2004 at the age of 25. He completed basic training at Fort Sill, Oklahoma, and advanced individual training at Fort Sam Houston, Texas. He became a Medic, and afterwards attended airborne training. When he was killed, he was assisting Soldiers injured by a bomb that had exploded a few minutes earlier.

Dustin is survived by his parents, David and Margaret; and his brother, Zack.

ROWAN D. WALTER

Died: February 23, 2007
Branch: U.S. Army

Private First Class Rowan D. Walter paid the ultimate sacrifice in service to his country on February 23, 2007, when he succumbed to wounds suffered on February 22 when an improvised explosive device detonated near his Humvee during combat operations in Ramadi, Iraq. The 25-year-old Medic served with the 1st Battalion, 9th Infantry Regiment, 2nd Brigade Combat Team, 2nd Infantry Division out of Fort Carson, Colorado. Two other Soldiers perished alongside him. A dedicated Medic to the end, Walter had left his vehicle to assist Soldiers wounded in an earlier attack. Private Walter was buried with full military honors in Clovis Cemetery, Clovis, California.

Rowan is survived by his wife, Priscilla; his parents, Bryan and Adele; his sisters, Hailey and Hanni; and his brother, Rome.

DAVID L. WATSON

Died: September 22, 2007
Branch: U.S. Army

Corporal David L. Watson died on September 22, 2007. He served as a Medic with the 2nd Battalion, 23rd Infantry Regiment, 4th Stryker Brigade, 2nd Infantry Division out of Fort Lewis, Washington. Watson died when he succumbed to non-combat related injuries in Baghdad, Iraq. He touched so many lives that his funeral had to be held in a high school auditorium to accommodate everyone. He was buried with full military honors at New Hope Cemetery in Jonesboro, Arkansas.

David is survived by his wife, Lisa; two sons, Dayton and David; his mother, Linda; two brothers, Bryant and Dereck; and two sisters, Chrystal and Nikki.

NATHAN L. WINDER

Died: June 26, 2007
Branch: U.S. Army

Green Beret Sergeant First Class Nathan L. Winder perished on June 26, 2007, from wounds sustained from enemy small-arms fire in Ad Diwaniyah, Iraq. The 32-year-old Special Forces Soldier had been assisting a quick reaction team engaged in combat. He was assigned to C Company, 2nd Battalion, 1st Special Forces Group, Fort Lewis, Washington, serving in support of Operation Iraqi Freedom as a member of the Combined Joint Special Operations Task Force. His family held a memorial service in his honor on July 6, 2007, at the North Latter Day Saints Chapel in Blanding, Utah. He was buried in Arlington National Cemetery, on July 13, 2007, with full military honors.

Nathan is survived by his wife, Michelle; his son, Logan; his parents Terri and Tom; and 14 siblings.

JONATHAN D. WINTERBOTTOM

Died: May 23, 2007
Branch: U.S. Army

Corporal Jonathan D. Winterbottom gave his life for his country on May 23, 2007, in Al Nahrawan, Iraq, when an IED hit his vehicle. Winterbottom, just a week shy of his 22nd birthday, was serving as a Medic with the 3rd Squadron, 1st Cavalry Regiment, 3rd Brigade Combat Team, 3rd Infantry Division out of Fort Benning, Georgia. Winterbottom is buried next to his mother in Oakwood Cemetery in Falls Church, Virginia.

Jonathan is survived by his father, Robert; his daughter, Lilly; his sister Sarah; and his brother, J.J.

JOSHUA R. ANDERSON

Died: January 2, 2008
Branch: U.S. Army

Private First Class Joshua R. Anderson died following the detonation of an improvised explosive device on January 2, 2008, in Kamasia, Iraq. A Combat Medic, Anderson was assigned to the 6th Squadron, 8th Cavalry Regiment, 4th Brigade Combat Team, 3rd Infantry Division out of Fort Stewart, Georgia, in support of Operation Iraqi Freedom. The 24-year-old Medic had been serving in Iraq for only two months prior to his death. He is buried at the Fort Snelling National Cemetery in Minneapolis, Minnesota. Joshua's acts of selfless service, so typical of his approach to life, will live forever in the hearts of his family and friends.

Joshua is survived by his wife, Hannah; his daughter, Savannah; his parents, Keven and Lynn; and his siblings, Michael and Jennifer.

RICHARD J. BERRETTINI

Died: January 11, 2008
Branch: U.S. Army

Lieutenant Colonel Richard J. Berrettini died on January 11, 2008, from injuries sustained when an IED hit his Humvee on his way back to his home base from the Khowst Province in Afghanistan. The attack occurred on January 2, and he was evacuated by air from Afghanistan through Landstuhl, Germany, to Brooke Army Medical Center in San Antonio, Texas. A dedicated Army Nurse Corps Officer, Richard was the first Army Nurse to die in Afghanistan, the third to die in the Global War on Terrorism. On January 18, 2008, a Mass of Christian Burial was celebrated at Our Lady of Mount Carmel Church in Pittston, Pennsylvania. He was buried with full military honors at the Mount Olivet Cemetery in Wyoming, Pennsylvania.

Richard is survived by his wife, Jane; his sons, Vincent and Christopher; his mother, Doris; and his brother, Nello.

ALBERT BITTON

Died: February 20, 2008
Branch: U.S. Army

Corporal Albert Bitton died on February 20, 2008, in Baghdad, Iraq, from injuries sustained while riding in a Humvee that encountered an improvised explosive device. He was 20 years old and had been serving in combat for seven months with the 1st Battalion, 502nd Infantry Regiment, 2nd Brigade Combat Team, 101st Airborne Division in support of Operation Iraqi Freedom. Hundreds of friends and family crowded inside Congregation Adas Yeshurun Synagogue in West Rogers Park community of Chicago, Illinois, on February 26, 2008, to honor his memory. He was buried at Memorial Park Cemetery, Skokie, Illinois.

Albert is survived by his wife of just a few months, Melissa; his parents, Elie and Silvia; and two sisters, Jackie and Elizabeth.

DUSTIN K. BURNETT

Died: June 20, 2008
Branch: U.S. Navy

United States Navy Corpsman Dustin K. Burnett was killed on June 20, 2008, in the Farah Province of Afghanistan, when his vehicle was hit by an improvised explosive device. The 19-year-old was with the First Marine Division out of Twentynine Palms, California. At the time of his death, Burnett had been serving in Afghanistan for three months in support of Operation Enduring Freedom. On July 4, 2008, Burnett's ashes were interred at the Riverside National Cemetery in Riverside, California, with full military honors.

Dustin's casket traveled through Dover Air Force Base and arrived in Bullhead City, Arizona, in the company of a military escort. Dustin's remains continued on to their final destination accompanied by an honor guard consisting of the Bullhead City Police, the Patriot Guard Riders, and state troopers. As the procession moved down the road, motorists pulled off the road, stopped, and paid silent homage to Dustin.

Dustin is survived by his parents, Donald and Debbie; and his brother, Devin.

ANTHONY CARBULLIDO
Died: August 8, 2008
Branch: U.S. Navy

Navy Petty Officer Second Class Anthony Carbullido was killed on August 8, 2008, in Sangatesh, Afghanistan, when his convoy was hit by an improvised explosive device. The 25-year-old Corpsman was working as an instructor at the Navy Hospital Corps School in Great Lakes, Illinois, when he was deployed to Afghanistan with the 1st Supply Battalion, Combat Logistics Regiment 15, 1st Marine Logistics Group. He was buried with full military honors at Guam Veterans Cemetery in Piti, Guam, on the day after what would have been his 26th birthday.

Tony is survived by his wife, Summer, and his daughter, Lexie; his parents, Anthony and Aurora; his brother, Austin; and his sister, Ashley.

RYAN J. CONNOLLY
Died: June 24, 2008
Branch: U.S. Army

Sergeant Ryan J. Connolly was killed on June 24, 2008, in Khogyani, Afghanistan, when a land mine exploded under his vehicle. Even though he was mortally wounded, he directed others in efforts to save the lives of fellow Soldiers. The 24-year-old Soldier served with the 173rd Special Operations Troops Battalion out of Bamberg, Germany. He was buried with full military honors in Santa Rosa Memorial Park in Santa Rosa, California. Hundreds of mourners lined the streets as his funeral procession made its way to the cemetery.

Ryan had a passion for baseball, classic muscle cars, and NASCAR racing. During his leave in April 2008, he had purchased a 1970 Chevy Nova and was excited about restoring it.

On one occasion, Connolly was one of the first Medics on the scene of a suicide bombing. He was credited with saving 17 Afghans.

Ryan is survived by his wife, Stefanie and their daughter, Kayla; his parents, James and Robin; his brother, Mike; and his sister, Kelly.

JESSICA A. ELLIS
Died: May 11, 2008
Branch: U.S. Army

Corporal Jessica A. Ellis was killed on May 11, 2008, when an improvised explosive device detonated near her vehicle in Baghdad, Iraq. The 24-year-old Medic was serving with the 2nd Brigade Special Troops Battalion, 2nd Brigade Combat Team, 101st Airborne Division out of Fort Campbell, Kentucky. She was buried in Arlington National Cemetery with full military honors. A funeral mass was held at St. Francis Cathedral in Baker City, Oregon. As a testament to her impact on her platoon, her Battalion Commander, Lieutenant Colonel Miguel B. Hobbs, and her Platoon Sergeant, Sergeant First Class Joseph Johnson, traveled from their posts in Iraq for the service. More than 300 of her fellow Soldiers also held a memorial service in Iraq.

Jessica leaves behind her parents, Steve and Linda; her brother, Cameron; and her sister, Mandy.

ERROL M. JAMES
Died: August 4, 2008
Branch: U.S. Army

Army Sergeant Errol M. James died on August 4, 2008, from injuries sustained at Forward Operating Base Torkham, Afghanistan. The 29-year-old Sergeant was a member of the 527th Military Police Company based out of Grafenwoehr, Germany. He was remembered by his military comrades in a ceremony held at Katterbach, Germany, where he had lived since October 2004. Sergeant James was buried in St. Croix, U.S. Virgin Islands, following a funeral at Fredensberg Church in Estate Glynn, St. Croix. He was laid to rest with full military honors.

A long and winding road brought Errol from his homeland far from American soil to his post as a Sergeant in the United States Army. Described by his friends as "dependable, loving and easygoing," Sergeant James was born in Antigua in 1979. He moved with his family to Anguilla at age 12 and after graduating from high school, he relocated to the island of St. Croix, where he enlisted in the United States Army in 2000.

Errol is survived by his wife, Eva; his son, Elijah; his mother, Jermaine; and his sister, Josette.

JANELLE F. KING
Died: August 14, 2008
Branch: U.S. Army

Army Private Janelle F. King died in Baghdad, Iraq, on August 14, 2008, while serving in Operation Iraqi Freedom. The 23-year-old was serving as a Medic with the 115th Combat Support Hospital from Fort Polk, Louisiana. She was stationed at Camp Cropper, a military detainee center near Baghdad International Airport, at the time of her death. Private King was buried at Fort Sill Post Cemetery in Lawton, Oklahoma.

King followed in the footsteps of her parents when she enlisted in the Army in May 2007. Her father, Brian, is an officer in the Air Force, and her mother spent a decade in the Air Force as well.

King is survived by her parents, Jamecia and Brian.

WILLIAM L. MCMILLAN, III
Died: July 8, 2008
Branch: U.S. Army

Specialist William "Bill" McMillan was serving in Abu Ghraib, Iraq, when he gave his life for his country on July 8, 2008. He was assigned to the 1st Battalion, 21st Infantry Regiment, 2nd Stryker Brigade, 25th Infantry Division out of Hawaii. He died 12 hours after an improvised explosive device struck the vehicle he was riding in. Funeral services were held for the 22-year-old Medic at Southland

Christian Church on July 19, 2008. Seven Army Black Hawk Helicopters performed a flyover at his funeral.

Bill is survived by his wife, Elizabeth; his parents, General William L. McMillan, Jr., and Marge McMillan; his brother, Bradley; and his sister, Lauren.

JOHN P. PRYOR
Died: December 25, 2008
Branch: U.S. Army

United States Army Reserve Major and Medical Corps Officer Dr. John P. Pryor died on December 25, 2008, of wounds incurred when a single mortar round hit his quarters in Mosul, Iraq. He served as a Physician in support of Operation Iraqi Freedom. A Mass of Christian Burial was celebrated for Major Pryor at the Cathedral Basilica of Saint Peter in Philadelphia, Pennsylvania. The internment took place on January 5, 2009, with full military honors. Before his final deployment, Major Pryor organized his own funeral rites, chose music to be played at the service, selected a casket, and composed his obituary to mitigate his family's burden in the event of his death.

He is survived by his wife, Dr. Carmela Calvo; and his three children, Francis Xavier, John, and Danielle.

JEFFREY M. RADA MORALES
Died: June 29, 2008
Branch: U.S. Army

Sergeant First Class Jeffrey M. Rada Morales, a 32-year-old member of the Green Berets, died June 29, 2008, in Sofla, Afghanistan. The brave Medical Sergeant was supporting his country in Operation Enduring Freedom when the vehicle he was riding in rolled into a canal and he and two of his comrades drowned. Sergeant First Class Morales was assigned to the 1st Battalion, 7th Special Forces Group out of Fort Bragg, North Carolina. He is buried in the Puerto Rico National Cemetery in Bayamon, Puerto Rico.

Jeff is survived by his wife, Amanda; his children, Jessica and Andrew; and his mother, Virginia.

GERARD M. REED
Died: June 11, 2008
Branch: U.S. Army

Sergeant First Class Gerard M. Reed died in Baghdad, Iraq, on June 11, 2008, while serving with the 86th Combat Support Hospital out of Fort Campbell, Kentucky. The 40-year-old Army Medic died from injuries he sustained in a non-combat related incident. Family and friends paid their final respects at Greater Missionary Baptist Church in Clarksville, Tennessee, and he was buried in Kentucky Veterans Cemetery West in Hopkinsville, Kentucky.

Gerard is survived by his wife, T'Wona; his son, Isaiah; his mother, Bobby; his father, Clyde; and his brothers, Jimmy and Cedric.

MARC A. RETMIER
Died: June 18, 2008
Branch: U.S. Navy

Navy Hospital Corpsman Marc A. Retmier died on June 18, 2008, from wounds he suffered during an enemy rocket attack in northern Paktika Province, Afghanistan. Retmier was treating local civilians when Taliban insurgents ambushed him. A comrade also died in the attack. The 19-year-old Sailor was serving with the Provincial Reconstruction Team in support of Operation Enduring Freedom. He was buried next to his uncle for whom he was named, also a 19-year-old member of the Navy, who died of natural causes while serving his country in 1975.

Marc is survived by his parents, Steven and Joy; and two younger brothers, Matthew and Mason.

ANDREW J. SHIELDS
Died: May 31, 2008
Branch: U.S. Army

Private First Class Andrew J. Shields died on May 31, 2008, on a hot dusty road near Jalalabad City, Afghanistan. An improvised explosive device detonated near the 19-year-old's vehicle. Shields served with the 173rd Special Troops Battalion out of Bamberg, Germany. He is buried in the Evergreen Memorial Gardens in Vancouver, Washington. Hundreds attended the funeral at New Heights Church in Vancouver. Two fire trucks were present; they extended and crossed their ladders. From scaffolding the firefighters suspended a full-size American flag.

Andrew is survived by his father, Jon; his mother, Wendy; his sister, Ryleigh; and his fiancée, Loren.

DAVID S. STELMAT, JR.
Died: March 22, 2008
Branch: U.S. Army

Sergeant David S. "DJ" Stelmat, an Army Medic serving with the 1132nd Military Police Company, died on March 22, 2008, in Baghdad, Iraq. The vehicle he was riding in was struck by an improvised explosive device. A mass was celebrated for David on March 28, 2008, in Centerville, Ohio.

David is survived by his mother, Maryanne; his father, David; three sisters; and his brother.

EICHMANN A. STRICKLAND
Died: September 9, 2008
Branch: U.S. Navy

Petty Officer Third Class Eichmann A. Strickland died on September 9, 2008, while serving in Afghanistan during Operation Enduring Freedom. Strickland was killed when the vehicle he was driving encountered an improvised explosive device in Kabul, Afghanistan.

He was 23 years old at the time of his death. His funeral took place at Northshore Christian Church in Everett, Washington, and he was buried at Cypress Lawn Memorial Park.

Strickland is survived by his parents, Ken and Yolanda; his brother, Nick; and many friends and family.

TIMOTHY H. WALKER
Died: November 8, 2008
Branch: U.S. Army

Staff Sergeant Timothy H. Walker fell victim to a makeshift bomb that detonated near his vehicle on November 8, 2008. He was serving in Baghdad, Iraq, in support of Operation Iraqi Freedom, and was within one month of completing his second tour in Iraq. At the time of his death, he was assigned to HQ Company, 64th Brigade Support Battalion, 3rd Brigade Combat Team, 4th Infantry Division out of Fort Carson, Colorado. The unit's mission in Iraq was to secure Sadr City in Baghdad's northeast sector. A memorial service was held in Sergeant Walker's honor at the Soldier's Memorial Chapel on Fort Carson on November 16, 2008.

Staff Sergeant Walker was a devoted family man, a benevolent human being, and a fine Soldier. His character was described as "loving, caring, and dedicated to his family and friends." He cared for his troops as he cared for his family, ever present and supportive.

Gordon Beck was Sergeant Walker's First Sergeant in the year 2000 at the 4th Engineer Battalion. He wrote that Sergeant Walker "took over a troubled Aid Station and quickly brought it up to snuff. He was a great medic and fine NCO."

Timothy is survived by his wife, Dawn, and his children, Gregory and Madison; his father, Wayne; and his mother Barbara.

CHRISTOPHER J. WEST
Died: February 4, 2008
Branch: U.S. Army

Corporal Chris J. West, a 26-year-old Combat Medic, died on February 4, 2008, at the 332nd Air Force Theater Hospital in Balad, Iraq, of wounds sustained a day earlier in Muqdadiyah, Iraq. West was assigned to the 1st Squadron, 73rd Cavalry Regiment, 82nd Airborne Division out of Fort Bragg, North Carolina. Family gathered to bury West on February 20, 2008, with full military honors, at Arlington National Cemetery.

He is survived by his parents, John and Hattie; his older sister, Lauren; and his younger sister, Cameron

JUSTIN R. WHITING
Died: January 19, 2008
Branch: U.S. Army

Staff Sergeant Justin R. Whiting died for his country on January 19, 2008, while he was on patrol near Mosul, Iraq, when the vehicle he was riding in was hit by an improvised explosive device. Staff Sergeant Whiting was assigned to the 3rd Battalion, 5th Special Forces Group based out of Fort Campbell, Kentucky. The Green Beret was serving his third tour in Iraq. Funeral services were held January 27, 2008, at the Hancock Central School auditorium, after which he was laid to rest with full military honors.

His younger brother, Nathan, who was also stationed in Mosul, Iraq, and who ate breakfast with Justin just hours before his death, remembers, "I got to see him that morning only by chance. We ate breakfast and then gave each other a hearty handshake and said goodbye, although we didn't know it was goodbye. He looked me in the eye and said, 'I'll see ya.' That's all, just 'I'll see ya.' Justin was a very simple man. He didn't put up with much, and you always knew how he felt. I never met anyone who was so determined."

Justin leaves behind his father, Randal; his mother, Estelline, his sister, Amanda; and his brother, Nathan.

EPILOGUE

This book has been a labor of love. Writing it has made me feel closer to these Soldiers, Sailors, and Airmen. My moto is: "If you are too big to do the little things, then you are too little to do the big things." The men and women in this book knew how to do the little things, which allowed them to do the BIG THINGS!!! May they Rest in Peace. I will never forget them.

- MSG (R) Matthew W. Sims
U.S. Army Combat Medic from 1997-2018
Three-time Purple Heart recipient.

EDITOR'S NOTE

What an honor to help to bring this author's work to the American public. This inspiring book moves one's soul to tears and triumph. My receiving this manuscript was an act of providence.

As an editor, author, and a multimedia journalist for the *Tri County Record* covering Berks, Chester, and Lancaster Counties, other sister papers, along with the Philadelphia suburbs in PA, I brought to life many stories of veterans and their organizations.

Working on this manuscript recalls a dear deceased family companion and friend, U.S. Army career Combat Medic SFC Harry J. Heater who served 1945-1969, World War II, Korean War, and Vietnam. This decorated hero earned a Combat Medical Badge with Star. He developed a love for my grandsons, Caleb and Joshua Quaintance (to whom he left a set of his dog tags). He taught them love of country and to honor all servicemembers with a "thank you for your service."

Harry and his son, Keith Heater (SFC ret.) took us all, along with my daughter-in-law Gloria Quaintance, and his daughters to tour Gettysburg and Washington, D.C., memorials on Memorial Day Weekend 2015. There he introduced us to his beloved "Jumping Mustang" buddies on their annual pilgrimage to "The Wall" and Arlington National Cemetery to honor their comrades who made the ultimate sacrifice.

May all who read this book celebrate Matthew Sims and all these heroes on the 250th Birthday of the U.S. Army and beyond.

- Carol Quaintance, Editor
(Mbr. of The Daughters of The American Revolution)

In celebration of all who fought in the Revolutionary War and for my dear Patriots, "Abraham Knerr and Philip Seyfert, blessed ancestors."

www.ingramcontent.com/pod-product-compliance
Lightning Source LLC
Chambersburg PA
CBHW050048080526
44586CB00014B/1519